REAL SOLUTIONS FOR ADULT ACNE

CURE HORMONAL ACNE WITH SCIENCE-BACKED TREATMENTS THAT WORK

KYLA STONE

PAPER MOON PRESS

Copyright © 2016 by Kyla Stone

All rights reserved. No part of this publication may be reproduced, distributed or transmitted in any form or by any means, including photocopying, recording, or other electronic or mechanical methods, without the prior written permission of the publisher, except in the case of brief quotations embodied in critical reviews and certain other noncommercial uses permitted by copyright law. For permission requests, write to the publisher, addressed "Attention: Permissions Coordinator," at the address below.

Paper Moon Press

Atlanta, GA/30328

This book is not intended as a replacement for professional medical care. It is not intended to diagnose, treat, prevent, or cure disease. Individuals should consult with their primary care physicians and dermatologists before taking any supplements or medications recommended in this book. While every effort has been made to present factual and up-to-date information, every fact in this book cannot be guaranteed. The author and publisher hold no responsibility for the consequences of following the plans and advice contained in this book.

Real Solutions for Adult Acne/ Kyla Stone —1st ed.

Printed in the U.S.A.

First Edition, May 2016

The text type was set in Gandhi Serif.

ISBN:978-1-945410-06-2

❃ Created with Vellum

To Jeremy. You have always supported me and believed in me on this journey.

CONTENTS

Acknowledgments	vii
Foreword	ix
Introduction	xi
Chapter 1	1
Chapter 2	5
Chapter 3	9
Chapter 4	12
Chapter 5	14
Chapter 6	18
Chapter 7	22
Chapter 8	28
Chapter 9	38
Chapter 10	47
Chapter 11	51
Chapter 12	56
Chapter 13	66
Chapter 14	75
Chapter 15	84
Chapter 16	89
Chapter 17	96
Chapter 18	98
Chapter 19	102
Chapter 20	109

Breakfasts	111
Lunches	117
Dinners	125
Snacks	135
Also By Kyla Stone	137
About the Author	139
References	141

ACKNOWLEDGMENTS

I would like to thank my beta readers and other members of my street team, including Derise Marden, Julie Muniz, and Nidhi Upadhyaya, for their dedication and hard work.

A huge thank you to all the dermatologists who took the time out of their busy schedules to lend their expertise to this book:

Dr. Sue Ellen Cox
Dr. Jeremy Brauer
Dr. David E. Bank
Dr. Elizabeth Tanzi
Dr. Vermén Verallo-Rowell
Dr. Debra Jaliman
Dr. Carol Trakimas
Dr. Peggy Fuller
Jennifer Waller
Laurie Thomas

FOREWORD

This book will help adults with acne, whether you develop acne following an acne-free adolescence, or you continue to develop acne recurrences from adolescence onward, or whether your acne suddenly begins again after years of being acne-free.

If your adult acne becomes more serious and you consult a dermatologist, *Real Solutions for Adult Acne* can help answer questions that weren't asked or even provide some ideas you may want to bring up with your dermatologist at the consultation.

At the same time, this book confirms, validates and re-enforces what your dermatologist will tell you. It also provides remedies above and beyond the traditional therapies prescribed in a dermatologist's office.

By following the advice in this book, you'll have less acne, less scarring and color changes post-acne, and your skin will look better — faster.

-Dr. Vermèn Verallo-Rowell

INTRODUCTION

I suffered from moderate to severe acne from the age of twelve until the age of thirty-two. I tried every prescription, every over-the-counter method, and every QVC miracle cream, but nothing worked. My acne negatively affected my self-esteem, my self-confidence, and my quality of life.

I struggled with depression and anxiety. I checked mirrors constantly—not because of vanity, but because I was worried that my concealer had worn off, that new pimples had popped up, and that my T-zone was an oil slick. I experienced anxiety every time I had to talk to someone up close and personal. Were they disgusted by my acne? Were they judging me?

There were times that I missed work or social occasions with friends because I was so ashamed of my skin. I was afraid to let anyone see me without makeup. Even now, I feel twinges of that old anxiety as I write this.

After years of experimenting with every expensive treatment

under the sun, I finally stumbled on a solution aimed at one of the major causes of adult acne—hormones. I researched hormonal treatments and convinced my dermatologist to let me try it.

I started on spironolactone in May of 2014. At the same time, I cleaned up my diet and avoided foods containing hormones, like meat and dairy.

By July, I was 95% clear. It changed my life.

My skin isn't perfect. Neither is my life. But the constant cloud of depression and anxiety has lifted. I can look in the mirror without hating what I see. And most importantly, I feel like I can be me again.

Are you ready to be free of that anxiety? Do you want to stop stressing over your skin and get on with your life?

It is my sincere hope that the information in this book will make a difference in your skin and in your life.

ONE

ADULT ACNE

"THERE IS STILL a common misperception that acne is just for teenagers," says Dr. Elizabeth Tanzi, founder and director of Capital Laser and Skin Care and assistant clinical professor of the Department of Dermatology at George Washington University Medical Center.

If only that were true! Unfortunately, adult acne is a pervasive problem. You are far from alone in your battle against adult acne. According to the *Journal of American Academy of Dermatology*, 54% of women age 25 and older suffer from acne. According to one study, 26% of women aged 31-40 had clinical acne, and 12% of women aged 41-50 had clinical acne.

While women are more likely to suffer from acne due to hormone fluctuations, men aren't exempt. According to a study from the University of Alabama, almost 43% of men in their twenties and 20% of men in their thirties still get acne. "This type of acne is primarily driven by male androgenic hormones," explains Dr. Vermèn Verallo-Rowell, a clinical and research dermatologist, dermatologic surgeon, and the author of over 150 articles on dermatology.

While both genders have androgens in their systems, men have more. A greater percentage of women have acne, but when men do get acne, it is usually worse. And research indicates that acne rates for both genders are rising.

Adult Acne is Different

Adult acne is different from the acne you suffered as a teen. In fact, some people have clear skin through their teen years and only develop acne as adults. The causes of adolescent acne and adult acne are slightly different. In adolescents, the sebaceous follicle responds to the rapid hormonal changes teenagers undergo by producing excess sebum.

Adult acne, while also hormonal, is triggered by different hormones, such as testosterone and stress hormones like steroids and cortisol. Adult acne is inflammatory. Acne is mostly on the face, particularly clustering around the mouth, chin, and jaw line. The pimples are large, deep, and red, rather than the fine bumps and blackheads many teenagers have.

As adults, we are more likely to have sensitive skin or combination skin. And in women, acne worsens with hormone fluctuations. You may notice acne flares around your period, pregnancy, and the onset of menopause. Conversely, some women experience clearer skin during pregnancy.

The causes of your adult acne are different from when you were a teen. And you can't use the same treatments you used as a teen and expect them to work the same way. They won't. Unfortunately, topical treatments tend not to work very well for adults. The root causes are deeper, and it takes a different approach to find the right solution that works for your adult skin.

The Emotional Effects of Adult Acne

As anyone who's suffered from acne for years knows by heart, acne is not just an annoyance or irritation. It can be debilitating to your happiness and self-esteem. It shouldn't be, but it is. People who've never experienced acne don't quite understand how painful it is to struggle with acne as an adult. The depression, the anxiety, and the stress can be overwhelming. A 2014 study found acne impacted sufferers as severely as those struggling with a chronic, debilitating disease.

The Answer

Too many articles in magazines simply tout the expensive products of companies that advertise with them. And they just don't work. While there isn't a 100% cure for acne, there is good news. Adult acne can be effectively managed through treatment and lifestyle changes.

This book will take you through the three major causes of adult acne and explore real treatments that get at the root of acne. Instead of just managing superficial symptoms, or doing nothing at all, you can eradicate your skin problems from the inside out.

You'll learn the most successful treatments for each cause,

including over-the-counter, prescription, and natural remedies you can make yourself. You'll get a diet plan with foods to eat and foods to avoid, as well as a Clear Skin Action Plan you can start today. This book also includes a seven-day jumpstart diet with recipes, a list of problem ingredients to avoid in your skincare products, a chapter on useful websites and resources, and a bibliography of the research cited in this book.

I've interviewed over a dozen experts in the field of dermatology. Each expert shares their best advice with you. I've also curated the best and most up-to-date research on what works and why. This book contains the tools you need to figure out the cause of your acne and aims to equip you with the resources you need to defeat your acne.

There is hope. You can live your life without obsessing over each new zit, without hating mirrors, without experiencing anxiety on a constant basis, and without wondering whether everyone in the room is staring at your skin.

While there is no 100% cure for adult acne, you can manage your acne successfully. The rest of this book will show you how.

TWO

THE SCIENCE OF ACNE

IF YOU'VE BEEN suffering from acne for years, you probably know more than you ever wanted to know about acne vulgaris. But I'll go over it quickly to make sure you're familiar with terms I'll use later.

Acne is a disease that involves the sebaceous and hair follicles of the skin. The sebaceous glands produce sebum (an oily substance that lubricates your skin) all over your body, but they are concentrated in your face and head. Normal amounts of sebum oil give you shiny hair and radiant skin. Too much leads to excessively oily skin.

The hair follicle acts like a wick, transporting the sebum and other cellular junk to the surface of the skin. These sebaceous glands are controlled predominately by the endocrine (hormonal) system. The sebaceous gland can become overactive due to puberty, hormonal fluctuations, stress, and heat and humidity. The follicles, or pores, become clogged due to the excessive sebum and buildup of dead skin cells. Bacteria thrive in this environment.

Acne is triggered by many different factors—or a combination of factors—in each individual person. However, the mechanism is the same across the board. The excess sebum, or oily secretions, in the sebaceous glands of the skin become infected with bacteria and dead skin cells that become trapped in the pores. Once the pores become inflamed, pimples, bumps, and cysts form.

ACNE FORMATION

There are different types of acne, according to the American Academy of Dermatology. Non-inflammatory acne includes blackheads and whiteheads. When oil, dead skin cells, and bacteria block pores, they can cause small bumps. If the pore stays open at the surface of the skin, the pore looks black and is called a blackhead. The black color is caused by the oil's reaction to the air. If a blocked pore closes up, the top of the bump looks white and is known as a whitehead.

TYPES OF ACNE PIMPLES

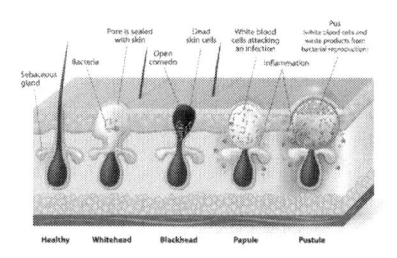

Inflammatory acne is deep, red, and painful. Inflammatory acne includes papules, pustules, nodules, and cysts. Papules are hard, red bumps. Pustules are filled with yellow puss. When the blocked pores get irritated further, they grow larger and deeper into the skin, forming hard nodules. Cysts are also large, but are puss-filled and softer.

Determine whether you inherited the tendency to develop acne, including cystic acne. If acne runs in the family on both sides, three out of four children are likely to suffer from it as well. While there is nothing you can do about genetics, you can do something about the other main causes of acne.

"Most people try to treat the skin externally as an independent organ and expect overnight results, but do nothing to treat the underlying problem," says Jennifer Waller, the founder and CEO of Celtic Complexion Luxury Skincare based in Raleigh, North Carolina.

You won't be able to slather on a miracle medication and expect miraculous results. Your skin is affected by a myriad of factors. "Treating acne effectively means attacking it from several angles," says Dr. Carol Trakimas, the medical director and president of the Dermatology Center in North Carolina.

The goal is threefold: to decrease the amount of bacteria by unclogging the pores, to decrease oil production by balancing hormones, and to minimize inflammation.

"You will never be free of acne simply by treating the surface of the skin," Waller warns. Topical treatments reach the symptom only—and not very effectively, either. To truly heal your skin, you need to look deeper.

THREE

THE MAIN CAUSES OF ADULT ACNE

THE MAIN causes of adult acne are hormonal, inflammatory, bacterial, and diet-related. This chapter provides a quick overview of each cause.

Bacterial

The only cause that can be treated topically is bacterial. The bacteria that cause acne, *P. acnes,* normally live harmlessly on the skin, but they flourish in the dark, oil-filled environment of clogged pores. *P. acnes* feed on grease and dead skin cells. They over-colonize and cause inflammation and acne. Topical applications like benzoyl peroxide help minimize lesions caused by these bacteria.

To reduce acne, you want to minimize bacterial growth as much as possible. I'll discuss how in chapter four.

Hormonal

Spikes in certain hormones such as testosterone cause excessive increases in sebum production. Increased oil leads to clogged pores and trapped bacteria, leading to big, fat zits. The stress hormone cortisol also activates oil production. More stress equals more pimples.

Some women also suffer from polycystic ovary syndrome (PCOS), a hormonal disorder characterized by irregular periods, excess hair growth, obesity, enlarged ovaries, infertility, and acne. Women with the disorder have high levels of testosterone.

Other women don't have elevated levels of testosterone, but they may be sensitive to the normal amounts of androgens in their system. Hormonal acne often causes flare-ups below the cheeks and around the chin and jawline. If your acne breaks out around your period or changes during pregnancy (either for better or worse), you might be a good candidate for hormonal treatment.

I'll discuss hormonal factors further in chapter five.

Inflammatory

Research has found a link between oxidative stress, or inflammation, and acne. In a 2012 study published in the *Journal of Drugs in Dermatology*, researchers found that inflammation and oxidative stress—caused by free radicals—can cause acne. The study found that decreased antioxidant levels, particularly vitamins A, C, and E, are commonly found in adults with acne. Studies have also found that people with acne have a higher burden of oxidative stress.

I'll discuss inflammation in more detail in chapter six.

Diet

Simple, refined carbs (think white bread and pasta) and simple sugars (candy, soda, donuts) spike your blood sugar levels. This triggers your skin's inflammatory response. Several studies have also found a link between acne and dairy products. Dairy and other animal-based products are injected with hormones, which make their way into our food. As we've already learned, our hormones control the sebum production in our sebaceous glands.

We'll examine diet in chapter seven.

FOUR

BATTLE YOUR BACTERIA

The P. acnes bacteria on the surface of your skin is one of the first causes of acne you want to target. You don't want to address the deeper issues when your makeup is still clogging your pores. The first step is to eliminate any products you are using or unhealthy habits that are causing bacteria to keep clogging your pores.

Certain hair and skin products can clog pores, ensuring a breeding ground for bacteria and making acne worse. Yes, you read that right. Your shampoo could be aggravating those pimples on your forehead. Hairspray and gel can also affect the skin around your hairline.

"Anything that touches the face on a regular basis can irritate and worsen acne," says Dr. Peggy Fuller, a board-certified dermatologist and founder of the Esthetics Center for Dermatology. Think about your cell phone, that scarf you haven't washed in two months, or a dirty baseball cap. She advises cleaning headsets, cell phones, and computer keys daily.

Check your bike helmet and "non-breathing" fabrics which can rub sweat, dirt, and oils into the pores during your work-out, recommends Dr. David E. Bank, dermatologist, Assistant Clinical Professor of Dermatology at Columbia Presbyterian Medical Center in New York, and author *of Beautiful Skin: Every Woman's Guide to Looking Her Best at Any Age.*

Wash your makeup brushes and sponges every day or every other day. Change your towels and pillowcases frequently. Try for at least twice a week or more.

The first tool in your acne arsenal should be an antibacterial topical application, like benzoyl peroxide or salicylic acid. If you've been to your dermatologist, a prescription like clindamycin may also help. I'll talk more about acne treatments beginning in chapter 10.

FIVE

MAKE YOUR MAKEUP WORK FOR YOU

Your Foundation, blush, moisturizer, and powder can all block pores and cause bacteria to fester. Sometimes the product irritates existing acne, rather than clogging the pores and directly causing acne. Make sure you check out the ingredients of all the products you use near and on your face, and change them out as necessary.

Once you've started treatment to heal the root causes of your acne, you want to make sure you aren't inadvertently triggering further pimple production through products that continue to clog your pores.

Problem Ingredients in Your Skincare Products

You can look for products labeled "non-comedogenic", but it won't help you much. This label alone doesn't mean it won't clog pores. Plenty of acne sufferers have discovered this the hard way. Unfortunately, you can't trust a product claiming to be non-comedogenic because there are no regulated standards for these statements. No matter what a product actually contains, a company can claim that it won't cause acne because there's no regulation or law stating they can't. It makes them money, and they don't have to prove it.

"Oil-free" isn't any better. Plenty of ingredients that aren't oils cause terrible breakouts. On the other hand, some oils are great for soothing acne-prone skin.

"Dermatologist-approved" is also a no-go. You have no way of knowing whether the dermatologist is on the cosmetic company payroll (many are). Such dermatologists are expected to approve every product.

Become an Acne Detective

Unfortunately, even ingredients in acne-fighting products can cause acne. I had to become an acne detective, examining every ingredient in every product I put on my face. You can do the same thing.

You can go to review sites, such as www.makeupalley.com and www.acne.org, to check whether certain products made other people break out. Makeup Alley reviews cosmetic products. Acne.org is great for researching the effectiveness of different acne treatments, which are reviewed by real people. They also have an excellent forum.

Check out the EWG's Skin Deep cosmetics database. It contains a database of 60,000 products and ingredients and scores them for toxicity. Unfortunately, the FDA doesn't regulate the cosmetic industry for safety either.

You can check your product's safety ratings yourself at www.ewg.org/skindeep.

You'll also want to look at the ingredients individually. Paula's Choice has a cosmetic ingredients dictionary that breaks up over 1500 cosmetic ingredients into poor, good, and best categories.

You can check it out at www.paulaschoice.com/cosmetic-ingredient-dictionary/.

Another great site is CosDNA (Cosmetic DNA), where you can search individual ingredients. You can also put the entire ingredients list in one search box. Many products have a list of their ingredients online which you can copy and paste. The website is www.cosdna.com.

In chapter 19, you'll find a list of common problem ingredients in cosmetics and skincare products. The list includes their comedogenic rating, courtesy of Sage Skin Care. They are graded on a scale of 0 to 5, with five being the most comedogenic (will definitely clog pores).

Avoid products with ingredients rated 3, 4, or 5 among the first eight ingredients. Product ingredients are listed in order of amount, such as water (20% of the product) down to, say, alcohol as the last ingredient (.05%). It is highly unlikely that you will be able to find products without any iffy ingredients at all. Choose products that either have none of these ingredients in the first eight listed items, or only one or two.

If you think a product is contributing to your acne, stop using it for several weeks and see what happens. "The bottom line is, listen to your skin," says Dr. Sue Ellen Cox, a dermatologic surgeon, a consulting associate professor at Duke University, and a RealSelf.com contributor.

It might take a while, but with a bit of sleuthing, you can find the right cosmetics and skincare products that won't cause your skin to break out.

SIX

BALANCE YOUR HORMONES

HORMONAL ACNE IS an androgenic disorder, meaning it is activated by the family of hormones called androgens. When it comes to acne, testosterone is the androgen in charge. While androgens are often considered male hormones, both men and women have active levels in their blood. A woman's level is usually a tenth of that found in men. This is why acne is often worse in men.

"Testosterone makes acne worse because the skin has androgen receptor cells," explains Laurie Endicott Thomas, a health and food expert and the author of *Thin Diabetes, Fat Diabetes: Prevent Type 1 and Cure Type 2*.

The testosterone in the bloodstream activates the sebaceous glands, increasing sebum production. The excess sebum clogs up the pores.

Estrogen

Both estrogen and testosterone bind to the cell receptors in the oil glands. When estrogen binds to the cell receptors, the estrogen "turns off" oil production and prevents acne. When estrogen levels fall, there is less estrogen to bind to the cell receptors. "The female hormone progesterone spikes and stimulates the oil glands, resulting in acne flare-ups before your period," explains Dr. Bank.

High Blood Sugar

High blood sugar also increases hormone production, which puts more testosterone into the bloodstream than is needed. Regulating your blood sugar helps regulate your hormones.

Stress

Stress is another source of hormonal acne. When you're stressed, your adrenal glands release testosterone into your blood stream.

Polycystic Ovarian Syndrome

The worst cases of acne in women of all ages, however, are usually associated with a condition known as Polycystic Ovarian Syndrome, or PCOS. PCOS results when insulin resistance leads to an imbalance of a woman's sex hormones, according to Thomas. These women have insulin imbalance, which stimulates the adrenal glands and leads to increased testosterone and the stress hormone cortisol. "This overload of male sex hormones may give them acne as well as masculine patterns of hair growth: they may have thinning hair on their heads and too much hair on their bodies and faces," says Thomas.

You can have hormonal acne without having an actual hormone imbalance that would show up on blood tests. Some women have normal testosterone levels in their blood, but they are extra sensitive to testosterone. Their body reacts with inflammation and overactive sebum production.

Signs of Hormonal Acne

You may have hormonal acne if your pimples are most active around your chin and jawline. Pimples are usually red, inflamed, and may be cystic.

Hormonal acne tends to produce deep and painful lesions. You may struggle with weight gain and excess hair growth (like under your chin).

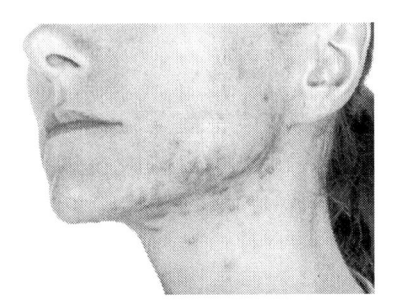

Hormonal acne is also resistant to topical treatments. This is because the problem is inside the body, not on the surface of the skin.

Treatments

Hormonal treatments block the effect of androgens on the oil glands, stopping acne before it begins. Hormonal acne is addressed with either birth control pills or an androgen-blocking medication such as spironolactone, or both.

Birth control pills work by altering estrogen levels. Most BCPs are a combination of synthetic estrogen and a synthetic progesterone compound known as progestin. A BCP brand containing more estrogen than progestin may lower the production of excess oils in the skin. Spironolactone works by blocking the androgen receptors.

Both spironolactone and BCPs are discussed in-depth in chapter 12 on prescription acne treatments. Many people, including myself, suffer for years and years, trying one thing after another to no avail. Antibiotics didn't help me. Retinoids didn't help me. Not even diet changes cleared me more than 50%.

Finally, I started looking into the hormonal cause of my persistent acne. Hormone therapy was a lifesaver for me, and for hundreds of thousands of others. I only wish I had access to the proper treatments earlier in my life. But at least I figured it out. And you will, too.

SEVEN

THE INFLAMMATION CONNECTION

CHRONIC INFLAMMATION IS a known factor in diabetes, heart disease, dementia, arthritis, stroke, cancer, asthma, dementia, and inflammatory bowel conditions like Crohn's Disease. Skin-wise, inflammation causes fine lines, dark circles, wrinkles, and chronic skin conditions such as dermatitis, psoriasis, eczema, and rosacea.

A 2013 study in *The Journal of Clinical and Aesthetic Dermatology* found that acne is an inflammatory disease. The authors cited histological, immunological, and clinical evidence suggesting that inflammation occurs at all stages of acne development.

So what causes inflammation?

The Stress Factor

The number one surprising reason you may have acne is

stress. "When your body is stressed, it releases cortisol, which signals the 'fight or flight' response. It also causes inflammation of the skin," says Waller.

"During stressful situations, your adrenal glands release more androgen hormones," says Dr. Trakimas. As we know from the last chapter, androgens stimulate excess oil production.

To lower stress and improve both your skin and your quality of life, incorporate stress-relieving techniques into your daily routine. Make sure you get seven to eight hours of sleep every night. Lower your daily intake of caffeine. Avoid alcohol, cigarettes, and drugs.

Exercise three to five times a week. A 2012 study found that middle-aged subjects who didn't exercise exhibited greater stress-related atrophy of the brain than people who exercised more.

Figure out your favorite ways to relax and work at least one into your schedule every day. Sit or lie down and just listen to music for 15 minutes. Practice yoga or meditation.

Go on a walk on a wooded nature trail or at a park. Get a daily dose of friendship by grabbing coffee (or better yet, a smoothie) with a friend. Tune in to your favorite stand-up comedian on Netflix and laugh yourself silly.

Finally, prioritize what's important and let the rest slide a little bit. Forgive yourself. Learn to say no to too many responsibilities. Take vacations. A balanced life benefits more than just your skin.

Your health—and your happiness—matter.

Medications

Certain drugs are also acnegenic, explains Dr. Verallo-Rowell. These include certain sleeping pills, antidepressants, and even some toothpastes and mouthwashes that contain fluoride.

Some medications can worsen acne. However, do not discontinue your medication if you suspect it's the cause of your breakouts. Talk to your doctor first. Maybe you can lower the dosage or switch to a similar medication.

Good and Bad Fats

"In addition to stress and/or medications, there are other factors that can cause inflammation. These include lack of sleep and a diet with an imbalance of omega-3 and omega-6 lipids," says Dr. Verallo-Rowell.

Long-chain omega-3 fatty acids include EPA (eicosapentaenoic acid) and DHA (docosahexaenoic acid). These are found primarily in fish and shellfish. Short-chain omega-3 fatty acids are ALA (alpha-linolenic acid). These are found in plants, like flaxseed. Though beneficial, ALA omega-3 fatty acids have less potent health benefits than EPA and DHA.

"In large amounts, omega-3s reduce the inflammatory process that leads to many chronic conditions," says Dr. Joseph C. Maroon in his book *Fish Oil: The Natural Anti-Inflammatory*. Many studies have documented the benefits of omega-3s at daily dosages between 2 and 5 grams of EPA and DHA.

Populations that consume the most omega-3 foods—like the people in Okinawa, Japan—tend to live longer and healthier lives than people who eat a standard diet low in omega-3s. The average Okinawa diet consists of fish and fresh produce. Researchers posited that Okinawans consume about eight times the amount of omega-3s than Americans on the standard American diet (SAD).

A 2008 study published in *Lipids in Health and Disease* showed that patients with acne taking 1000mg of omega-3 supplements for eight weeks experienced a marked improvement in their acne. Another small 2012 study in the same journal found fish oil appears to improve moderate to severe inflammatory acne (although the results did not apply to those with mild acne). And in 2014, Korean researches published a study that showed 2000 mg of omega-3 fatty acids taken daily for 10 weeks reduced inflammatory acne by 40% to 50%.

Omega-3s boast some awesome inflammation-reducing abilities. They support proper neurological function, maintenance of the cell membrane, mood regulation, and hormone production. Eat several servings a week from the sources listed below. You can also take fish oil supplements. Aim for 2000 to 3000 mg of omega-3s a day.

When choosing a fish oil supplement, look for high-quality wild, not farmed, salmon. Choose wild because farmed salmon has 20% more saturated fat as well as 5 to 10 times the amount of PCB pollutants, according to the Environmental Working Group (EWG).

Omega-3's:
    Salmon fish oil

4767 in 1 tbsp.
Cod liver oil
2664 mg in 1 tbsp.
Walnuts
2664 mg in ¼ cup
Chia seeds
2457 mg in 1 tbsp.
Flaxseed (ground)
1597 mg in 1 tbsp.
Hemp seeds
1000 mg in 1 tbsp.

To derive the most benefit from omega-3s, you also need to lower your intake of omega-6s. Today, we consume around 20 times more omega-6s than omega-3s.

Dr. Verallo-Rowell avoids any foods rich in the wrong kinds of fats. "These contain the omega-6 fats which are pro-inflammatory and also inflame the follicles in the skin," she says.

Excessive amounts of omega-6 fatty acids can promote inflammation, a key element in dozens of chronic diseases. Research shows that upping your omega-3s and reducing your omega-6s positively impacts every condition that has ties to inflammation.

You can eat less omega-6s by decreasing your use of oils such as soybean oil, corn oil, olive oil, margarine, shortening, most salad dressings, mayonnaise, and processed foods and snacks.

Case Study

Thirty-six-year-old Judy Marrow initially started taking omega-3 fish oil supplements at the recommendation of her eye doctor to treat her dry eyes. She'd struggled with adult acne for many years. After three months of taking fish oil, "my skin is so much clearer and I have less breakouts. I'm pretty much acne-free as long as I take omega-3 fish oil," she says. She still takes 1 1/2 tbsp. a night in liquid form.

EIGHT
YOU ARE WHAT YOU EAT

I KNOW YOU don't want to hear it. I know I didn't. I wanted a magical cure that would be easy, that wouldn't require much work or sacrifice. Unfortunately, that isn't the case. Expert opinions on whether diet affected acne seesawed for years. First, chocolate and pizza could make you break out. Then, it didn't matter what you ate.

Over the last several years, researchers have dug deeper. In 2010, a massive review of 50 years of clinical studies found a definitive link between diet and acne, after all.

Nonwestern populations do not experience acne like we do. A 2001 study published in the *Journal of the American Medical Association Dermatology* found zero incidents of acne in over 1000 research subjects in the non-westernized populations of the Kitavan Islanders of Papua New Guinea and the Ache hunter-gatherers of Paraguay. The researchers concluded that environment must play a role in acne development. Both these populations subsist on a plant-based diet devoid of processed or refined foods.

It is our typical western diet of refined sugars, refined carbs, fake sweeteners, and genetically modified foods that are wreaking havoc on our skin. Numerous studies have found that eating foods with a high glycemic index (GI) and consuming dairy and processed foods aggravate acne.

The good news is we can change our diet. However, altering your diet probably won't clear your skin completely, since diet is only one of the causes of acne. "Not everyone improves from dietary changes," warns Dr. Tanzi. But enough people do think it is worth trying. Many people see marked improvement when they cut problem foods out of their diet. For some people, it's refined carbs. For others, it's dairy. And for still others, it's both.

Ditch the Dairy

Many Americans eat a diet rich in refined carbs, unhealthy fats, and hormone-filled animal products. Meat and dairy both contain the animal's hormones, which affect humans, too. "Dairy causes spikes in certain pimple-producing hormones," says Dr. Trakimas. Dairy products also contain growth hormones which can exacerbate acne flares.

"Dairy foods are a big source of estrogen," explains Thomas. She describes how a diet high in animal-protein causes the liver to produce a powerful hormone called insulin-like growth factor-1 (IGF-1). IGF-1 activates the growth of the cells inside pores. The extra oil and the extra skin cells that shed into the pores produce acne. "The casein protein provokes the liver to produce the excess IGF-1 that causes overgrowth of the cells that line the pores," she says.

"If you remove the fats and the animal hormones and animal protein from the diet, the acne usually goes away by itself," says Thomas. She agrees that dairy is a major acne instigator. Switching to organic won't help either. Organic milk still contains estrogens because cows are milked while they are pregnant.

"The exact relationship between dairy—especially milk—and acne is unknown," says Dr. Cox. Some people can drink five glasses of milk a day and their skin is clear all day long. Others are sensitive to the hormone load and can't handle even small amounts.

A study conducted by the Harvard School of Public Health found a definitive link between milk drinkers and their acne. "Casein, the protein found in dairy products, produces an allergic response in many people," says Waller. "The immune system reacts by trying to fight the perceived toxin, and excess inflammation is produced." As we've learned, inflammation usually equals acne.

Avoid High Glycemic Foods

We know by now that high glycemic index (GI) carbohydrates like white bread, donuts, chips, and candy bars are bad for the waistline. But they have another dark side. Because they are absorbed into the blood stream so quickly, high GI foods raise blood sugar and insulin levels. The shot of excess insulin promotes inflammation and contributes to diabetes, heart disease, several cancers—and acne. This process also triggers a boost in androgen levels.

Scientists believe high GI foods directly affect acne because the hormone fluctuations activate an increase in sebum production. One 2007 Australian study found men on a strict, low GI diet noticed a dramatic improvement in their acne. Low GI foods like whole grains and vegetables don't trigger hormone spikes and don't aggravate acne.

The glycemic index ranks foods on a scale of 1 to 100 as a measure of how quickly the carbohydrate in the food is broken down and absorbed into the bloodstream. So what is considered high?

- High: 70-100
- Medium: 56-69
- Low: 55 or less

The higher the rise in glucose (sugar), the more insulin must be produced to store it. Higher insulin levels over time results in inflammation, elevating hormones which stimulate the activity of your oil glands. Sound familiar? Inflammation and hormone spikes are a vicious cycle.

Acne is rare in populations that eat diets with low glycemic values (and little to no dairy), according to several studies. Similar results have been replicated in the United States when subjects change their diets. A University of Miami study looked at the acne of 1900 volunteers on the low glycemic "South Beach" diet. More than 80% of participants saw improvement in their acne within three months.

Gut Bacteria and Acne

More than 2000 years ago, Hippocrates said, "All disease begins in the gut." More and more research is proving his hypothesis correct, at least in regards to acne. A healthy gut flora consists of hundreds of species of microorganisms. Good bacteria play an essential role in a healthy immune system. Good gut flora does the following:

- Helps to break down food
- Reduces inflammation
- Heals and repairs the lining of the intestinal wall
- Helps to shuttle out toxins from the body
- Keeps yeast growth and pathogenic microbes in check

Healthy gut flora can be negatively altered via antibiotics (which are often taken for acne) and a diet high in refined sugars, simple carbs, and other processed foods. Sanitizers and frequent washing of both hands and surfaces eliminates the intake of environmental bacteria, which helps to repair damaged gut flora.

We all have good and bad bacteria in our digestive system. When the gut flora is in balance, the bad bacteria (like E.coli) don't pose a threat to our health. But when bad bacteria outweigh the good, irritation and systemic inflammation throughout the body—and skin—occurs.

Dysfunctional gut flora leads to systemic inflammation and oxidative stress, both of which we've already learned activates the hormones that lead to acne. "When the good and bad bacteria in the gut are out of balance, it negatively affects the entire system," says Waller.

In a 2008 study published in *Clinical Gastroenterology and Hepatology,* inappropriate growth of bacteria in the small intestine was ten times more prevalent in people with acne than in healthy controls. A 2001 study conducted in Russia found that 54% of study participants with acne had an overabundance of bad bacteria in their gut.

A 2011 study found a link between gut microbes and acne. The researchers hypothesized that an imbalance in gut microbes had an effect on inflammation, oxidative stress, glycemic control, lipid levels, and bacteria.

How can you add beneficial bacteria to your gut? First, eat fresh vegetables and plenty of plant products (same as the low-glycemic diet!) and take a quality probiotic.

Probiotics are full of good bacteria, which can help restore a healthy balance in your gut. Probiotics stimulate the development of the gut and immune system. A good probiotic can help with any gut bacteria issues. Waller recommends Dr. Ohhirra's Probiotics, available at Whole Foods.

The Elimination Diet

So how can you tell what foods are triggers for you? Usually it's not a specific food, like chocolate, but a group of foods, like refined sugars, refined carbs, and/or dairy. For me, cutting out dairy for three months reduced my acne by 50%. You'll have to experiment to see what works for you.

Thomas recommends a low-fat, vegan diet. "It will improve your overall health while it makes you pretty," she says. I do recommend trying a vegan diet for at least twelve weeks. Cutting out dairy while continuing to eat meat, or vice versa, will defeat your efforts, since both meat and dairy contain the excess hormones you're trying to eliminate.

And remember, acne begins forming weeks and months before it erupts from your chin. Trying a diet for two weeks isn't going to reveal your underlying acne triggers. If you eat a piece of pizza and find a new zit the next day, the pimple wasn't from the pizza. It's not about individual meals; acne is a deeper, systemic issue.

When you start your diet, you want to eliminate all dairy and to eat healthy, low-GI foods for twelve weeks. Don't quit early. Commit to the full twelve weeks, minimum. And monitor your results. See how your skin looks. Keep a diary. Keep track of the number and severity of your pimples and cysts on a weekly basis.

Once you've cleared out your system and found your baseline, you can loosen up a bit. Often, you will find that you can add back small amounts of the forbidden food. I found I could eat up to two servings of cheese or yogurt a week and maintain the improvements in my skin. More than that, and I started to break out again. "Once people see the beautiful changes in their skin, they rarely return to their old habits," Waller says.

What to Eat

Low-glycemic doesn't mean low carb. It means eating

healthy carbohydrates. Think steel cut oatmeal (not instant), quinoa, sweet potatoes, lentils, beans, and 100% whole wheat pasta. While pasta is often lumped into the "bad foods" category, it shouldn't be. When pasta is cooked *al dente* (barely tender) and eaten in moderation, it doesn't negatively affect the body's glycemic load.

In general, you want to eat whole grains, fruits, and vegetables. Whole grains that will keep your blood sugar stable include quinoa (53), barley (28), bulgur (48), whole wheat grains (range from 30-54), and brown rice (50). Longer cooking times and further refining increase the glycemic index. While steel cut oatmeal is around 50, instant oatmeal comes in as high as 83.

You want to avoid processed foods like boxed cereals, crackers, rice cakes, instant oatmeal, baked goods, candy, white bread, white rice, and white potatoes. For example, white bread can be as high as 80, and white rice as high as 89.

Remember, it's all about balance and common sense. Think natural, unprocessed, unrefined foods, and you'll be fine. Carrots are high on the glycemic index at 71, but you certainly shouldn't stop eating them.

What About Protein?

You may worry about your protein intake on a healthy, low-fat, vegan diet. Most of us think of meat and dairy as the primary contributors of protein in a healthy diet. If you take out those foods, then how will you get enough protein? "The fear of protein deficiency is total nonsense," claims Thomas.

"We have known since the early 20th century that human

beings can easily meet their protein requirements on a purely plant-based diet," she says. "As long as you get enough calories, the protein will take care of itself." According to Thomas, there are no studies showing protein deficiencies in vegans as long as subjects ate sufficient calories.

The American Dietary Recommendation (RDA) for protein is 0.36 grams per pound. For the average 140-pound woman, that's only 50 grams a day. According to the documentary *Forks Over Knives*, vegetarians and vegans actually average 70% more protein than they need every day.

You can easily get your daily requirements through a plant-based diet. Check out a few foods high in protein:

- Lentils, 1 cup cooked (18 grams)
- Black beans, 1 cup cooked (15 grams)
- Chick peas, 1 cup cooked (15 grams)
- Tofu, 4 oz. (10 grams)
- Quinoa, 1 cup cooked (8 grams)
- Peas, 1 cup cooked (8 grams)
- Peanut butter, 2 tbsp (8 grams)
- Spaghetti, 1 cup cooked (8 grams)
- Almonds, ¼ cup (8 grams)
- Soy milk, 1 cup (7 grams)
- Cashews, ¼ cup (5 grams)
- Spinach, 1 cup cooked, (4 grams)

"If you are following a vegan diet, you will need a B12 supplement," says Thomas. There are no plant-based sources of vitamin B12, but you can take a 10-microgram daily supplement or a 2000-microgram weekly supplement. The recommended ADA is 2.4 micrograms a day. Too little B12 can cause anemia or nervous system damage over time.

But that's it. Other than B12, every other nutritional need can be satisfied through a healthy vegan diet. As long as you're getting several servings of fruits, vegetables, and whole grains a day, you can meet all your nutritional needs. And don't think that vegan equals food that tastes bland or dry as cardboard. There are plenty of delicious, healthy, easy-to-make vegan meals you can try.

In chapter 20, titled Jumpstart Your Clear Skin Diet Plan, I've included a seven-day diet plan, complete with recipes for breakfast, lunch, dinner, and a daily snack to jumpstart your journey. Several of the recipes include pictures.

In the next chapter, we'll talk about antioxidants and other superfoods that promote healthy skin from the inside out.

NINE
COMBAT OXIDATIVE STRESS

I TALKED ABOUT inflammation in chapter seven, which is caused in major part by oxidative stress. Oxidation occurs when your body processes the oxygen you breathe in, and your cells create energy from it. This process also produces free radicals—molecules that interact with our cells, resulting in stress, or damage, to other cells and DNA. Free radicals are normal, but when too many free radicals are present, they overwhelm the repair process. This is known as oxidative stress.

Oxidation happens when our cells are making energy, when our immune system is fighting bacteria and creating inflammation, when we are physically and emotionally stressed, and when our bodies are working to detoxify pollutants such as pesticides, smoke, etc. Oxidative stress causes aging, grey hair, wrinkles, arthritis, muscle and joint pain, fatigue, headaches, cancer, and, of course, acne.

Reduce Oxidative Stress

There are two ways to reduce oxidative stress. The first way is to avoid exposure when possible. We avoid exposure when we minimize stress, avoid overexposure to UV rays, avoid toxins in our environment and in our food, and reduce our sugar and chemical intake.

The second way to reduce oxidative stress is to increase our intake of antioxidants. Antioxidants are chemicals that promote or slow cell damage. They block the oxidation process.

Acne sufferers are often particularly sensitive to oxidative stress. One study found that blood levels of antioxidant vitamins like A, C, and E are lower in people with acne compared to those without acne. A 2012 study published in *The Journal of Drugs in Dermatology* found that increasing antioxidant consumption reduces the amount of oxidative stress, which in turn reduces acne.

Eat Your Antioxidants

Antioxidants also reduce inflammation throughout the body. Get your antioxidants and other nutrients from real food, not from supplements or pills. You'll want to include plenty of fruits, vegetables, nuts, and herbs in your diet. Dr. Trakimas suggests trying to include as many anti-inflammatory superfoods in your diet as you can.

Remember, supplementing your diet with isolated, synthetic nutrients via pills affects the body very differently than when you consume the same nutrients from real food sources. You want to transform your skin from the inside out. Synthetic pills stuffed with massive amounts of super vitamins tend to lead to very expensive pee. In addition, supervitamins can sometimes do more harm than good.

For example, vitamin A is a fat-soluble vitamin, which means it builds up in the body. Taking a high-dose vitamin A supplement (above 10,000 IU) can lead to side effects such as blurred vision, dizziness, headaches, and loss of muscle coordination.

Simply eating your antioxidants is the healthier and more enjoyable option. You can easily incorporate the following lists of foods into your diet several times a week to supercharge each meal. You should see healthier, plumper, clearer skin within three months.

Top 20 Antioxidant Foods to Eat

- Goji berries
- Wild blueberries
- Red kidney beans (dried)
- Pinto beans
- Cranberries
- Artichoke (cooked)
- Blackberries
- Prunes
- Raspberries
- Strawberries

- Apples
- Pecans
- Sweet cherries
- Black plums
- Russet potatoes
- Black beans (dried)
- Plums
- Dark chocolate

Types of Antioxidants and Where to Find Them

- Allium sulphur compounds: Leeks, onions, garlic
- Anthocyanins: Eggplant, grapes, berries
- Beta-carotene: Pumpkin, mangoes, apricots, carrots, spinach, parsley
- Catechins: Red wine, tea
- Copper: Seafood, lean meat, milk, nuts, legumes
- Cryptoxanthins: Red peppers, pumpkin, mangoes
- Flavonoids: Tea, green tea, red wine, citrus fruits, onion, apples
- Indoles: Cruciferous vegetables such as broccoli, cabbage, cauliflower
- Lignans: Sesame seeds, bran, whole grains, vegetables
- Lutein: Corn, leafy greens (such as spinach)
- Lycopene: Tomatoes, pink grapefruit, watermelon

- Manganese: Seafood, lean meat, milk, nuts
- Polyphenols: Thyme, oregano
- Selenium: Seafood, offal, lean meat, whole grains
- Vitamin C: Oranges, berries, kiwi fruit, mangoes, broccoli, spinach, peppers
- Vitamin E: Vegetable oils, nuts, avocados, seeds, whole grains
- Zinc: Seafood, lean meat, milk, nuts

Top 10 Antioxidant Herbs

- Clove
- Cinnamon
- Oregano
- Turmeric
- Cocoa
- Cumin
- Parsley (dried)
- Basil
- Ginger
- Thyme

Top Super Foods that Heal and Renew Skin

Instead of focusing so much on what not to eat, try focusing on what you can eat. Try to include the superfoods listed below at least a few times a week. These foods aren't just antioxidant, low glycemic, or dairy-free; they are all three—and packed to the gills with ingredients that hit acne-plagued skin on several fronts.

Sweet Potatoes

Sweet potatoes are full of antioxidants. They're also rich in vitamins A and C, both known to play an important role in preventing and healing acne. Sweet potatoes are also low glycemic, unlike regular potatoes.

Oranges

Oranges have a ton of vitamin C, which helps the body produce more collagen and elastin, promoting radiant, even skin tone. Oranges are also rich in vitamin A, one of the most important nutrients for healthy skin.

Peppers

Red, yellow, and green peppers are spiked with Vitamin C.

Garlic

Garlic is a potent antioxidant. It also contains a compound called allicin, which has antibacterial and anti-inflammatory properties.

Avocados

Avocados are full of B-complex vitamins, which are anti-inflammatory. They are rich in vitamins A, D, and E, all nutrients critical in the health and appearance of your skin. They are also delicious!

Green Leafy Veggies

Kale, chard, spinach, and collard greens are all high in manganese, which promotes collagen formation in skin cells—keeping your skin supple and youthful. Leafy greens are also abundant in Vitamin A, which lowers the amount of oil the sebaceous glands release. Add leafy greens to salads, omelets, soups, and sandwiches.

Coconut Oil

The medium chain fatty acids in coconut oil prevent oxidation. It also contains lauric acid, which is anti-bacterial, anti-fungal, anti-viral, and anti-inflammatory. Coconut oil can be used in cooking in place of your typical oil. It can also be used topically as a moisturizer.

Mushrooms

Mushrooms contain antioxidants and riboflavin (vitamin B2), which is used in the repair and maintenance of skin tissue. Shitake mushrooms in particular are a great source of kojic acid, which lightens age, sun, and acne spots.

Dark Chocolate

What you've heard is true. Dark chocolate (at least 75% cacao) is high in antioxidants and flavanols, which protect your skin from UV rays and improves skin texture, tone and hydration levels.

Almonds

Almonds are abundant in vitamin E, which protects against skin cancer, age spots, lightens dark circles and moisturizes skin. Vitamin E also fights inflammation.

Pumpkin Seeds

These seeds are rich in selenium (a potent antioxidant), vitamin E, essential fatty acids, and zinc. Zinc maintains collagen production. Research suggests zinc deficiency is associated with acne outbreaks. Try ¼ cup a day.

Ground Flaxseed

Flaxseed is a great source of omega-3s. Omega-3s reduce the appearance of wrinkles by softening and smoothing the skin. Fatty acids also reduce the inflammation that triggers our cells to clog pores. You also get omega-3s from fish oil supplements. Eat a tablespoon a day.

Green Tea

This tea is a potent inhibitor of inflammation. It also regulates testosterone production in women. Use loose tea leaves or powder instead of tea leaves to maximize EGCG, green tea's best acne fighting ingredient. Aim for two cups a day.

TEN

OVER-THE-COUNTER ACNE MEDICATION

OVER-THE-COUNTER (OTC) products can be tricky. It's hard to know what really works through all of the marketing hype and photoshopped advertisements. OTC acne products are generally for mild cases. If your typical products aren't working or your acne is moderate or severe, your best bet is to see a dermatologist. Remember, products like benzoyl peroxide attack bacteria, which is only one of the causes of acne. Topical OTC products should only be one part of your acne-fighting arsenal.

According to the Mayo Clinic, the top OTC products include benzoyl peroxide, salicylic acid, AHAs and BHAs, and sulfur. You always want to use the smallest amount that's effective.

Adult skin is easily irritated. If any of these products causes you to break out, return or discard them and keep looking for your holy grail skin care products.

Benzoyl peroxide

Benzoyl peroxide kills the *P. acnes* bacteria. OTC BP comes in strengths of 2.5% to 10%. Several studies have shown that the 2.5% version is just as effective at reducing acne without all the drying, irritating side effects.

However, too much benzoyl peroxide can cause scaliness, redness, burning, and stinging. Start with a small amount and work your way up. BP can bleach your towels and your clothes, so be careful when you use it.

BP is the main ingredient in the Acne.org regimen of choice. To try it, wash your face with a gentle cleanser. Wait for your skin to dry completely, about 15 minutes. Then apply 2.5% BP. Start with a pea-sized amount, but gradually work your way up to slathering on a full finger-length's worth. Gently massage into your skin for three minutes without rubbing. Wait another 5-15 minutes for the BP to fully absorb into your skin, then apply a liberal amount of moisturizer the same way, gently massaging into skin without rubbing. For more details on the Acne.org regimen, visit www.acne.org/regimen.

Salicylic Acid

Salicylic works by preventing pores from clogging by sloughing away dead skin cells. OTC strengths range from 0.5% to 5%. Because salicylic acid and benzoyl peroxide work differently, you can use them in combination to fight acne. You may decide to use benzoyl peroxide in the morning and salicylic acid at night, for example.

Alpha and Beta Hydroxy Acids

I'll talk about these acids more in chapter 14 on chemical peels. Some acids such as glycolic acid and lactic acid are also found in much lower concentrations in nonprescription products. They improve problem skin by removing dead skin cells, reducing inflammation, and stimulating the growth of new skin tissue.

AHAs can be found in lotions, washes, and night creams. They are low strength and safe to use up to twice a day, as long as it doesn't dry out your skin. I find I get better results with a weekly AHA peel.

Sulfur

Sulfur is usually combined with other ingredients like salicylic acid. It removes dead skin cells and excess oil off the surface of the skin. It is available in leave-on products such as spot treatments. It works best for targeted areas like individual pimples rather than all over your face.

Retinol

Retinol is a derivative of vitamin A and a weaker version of the prescription tretinoin, aka Retin A. It works by unclogging the pores and revealing fresher, more radiant skin. It's often found in anti-aging products as well. Both retinol and tretinoin can be very drying.

For mild acne, these over-the-counter remedies may work great, especially combined with the diet changes I've advised in previous chapters. For moderate and severe acne, topical OTC applications don't usually cut it. And if the cause is hormonal or inflammatory, you won't ever see the improvement you're looking for.

If this is your situation, don't delay any longer. Make an appointment to see a dermatologist. The right prescription medication can make all the difference in the health of your skin.

ELEVEN

SEE A DERMATOLOGIST, PRONTO

WHILE THE THOUGHT of using only natural products to clear your skin is appealing, the reality is that acne is persistent and pervasive. Sometimes you need strong tactics to do battle with a strong adversary. That's where a dermatologist comes in. Dermatologists have the knowledge and the experience to prescribe medications that can truly make a difference in your skin.

You might be surprised at how affordable it can be. Prescription acne products are usually covered by insurance. Many times, generic versions are available. And many aren't that expensive, especially considering the costs of various miracle creams and lotions touted by the next famous so-and-so that never seem to work as promised. "We see so many patients who have literally spent thousands of dollars on miscellaneous miracle treatments from blogs, QVC, or the Internet, all to no avail," says Dr. Fuller.

Debra Gordon of Milford, Connecticut, recommends doing

some of your own research before visiting your dermatologist. She struggled with acne for twenty-four years before clearing her skin with a combination of a vegan, low-glycemic diet and benzoyl peroxide. She used Acne.org to research treatment options and learn from others' experiences in the forums. "Take skin advice from well-meaning friends and family with a grain of salt," she adds. "Listen to the experts!"

At the same time, don't be afraid to ask questions about a treatment option you've read or heard about. I'm the one who brought up spironolactone to my dermatologist. I researched and advocated for myself. Once she saw my great results, she started prescribing the same treatment for some of her other patients.

Signs of a Good Doctor

You want a doctor who will listen to you and take your specific experiences into account. Dr. Verallo-Rowell sits down with her patients and asks a barrage of questions to uncover the triggers for each individual patient. She asks what they eat, what sports they play, what makeup they wear, what treatments they've tried, and what other conditions they struggle with. "A doctor who takes the time to look holistically at your history and lifestyle will be able to guide you through the different options," suggests Dr. Cox.

Look for a doctor with experience working with adult patients. You can't treat adult acne the same way you do adolescent acne. Dr. Fuller recommends finding a dermatologist with a special interest in nutrition as well as dermatology, and who is well versed in the latest breakthroughs in chemical peels, laser and light therapies, and scar minimizing. Adults are more likely to have hyperpigmentation and scarring due to dealing with acne for a decade or more.

Red Flags

Like many things in life, it might take some trial and error to find the right fit. Watch out for the following red flags. If the dermatologist doesn't take your history, that's a huge warning sign. The doctor should be asking about your family history, your allergies, and any other skin or health issues.

And if she isn't asking you about your current skin care regime, then she's not the doc for you. Your dermatologist should be asking you for details about everything you put on your face. Certain products could be drying you out or further irritating your acne. She also needs to make sure the medication she's going to prescribe for you is compatible with what you're currently using.

You also want to leave the doctor's office feeling confident about what your particular issues are, what medicine you'll be taking, and why. You shouldn't feel rushed or like you're receiving assembly line care. If the doctor didn't take the time to explain your diagnosis, treatment plan, or possible pros and cons, that's a problem.

Finally, if the dermatologist is giving you a hard sell about a certain procedure with his brand new laser or aggressively touting the skincare line he happens to carry in his office, that's another red flag. You and your health should be the top priority.

The Treatment Plan

Go into your treatment plan with realistic expectations. Nothing will heal acne overnight. Expect to give a good treatment plan three to six months before determining its effectiveness—or quitting prematurely. Sometimes, things get worse before they get better.

"Follow your doctor's advice to the letter," says Dr. Verallo-Rowell. Skipping treatments or taking shortcuts can affect your results—and not for the better. Adding other products or steps before you're clear can affect your results as well. If you add a new product and you start breaking out, it makes it harder to know what is working and what isn't.

It's important to remember that your experience won't mimic the results of someone else. Every individual is unique. "The best treatment is the one that works for you," says Dr. Cox.

Fitting It In

"If fitting in an appointment is too difficult with an adult's busy schedule, patients have the option to use a dermatology care service that's entirely online. We use DermatologistOnCall to see patients online and even for handling check-ups," explains Dr. Trakimas. Dermatologists can diagnose and prescribe a treatment plan, all online.

DermatologistOnCall is a network of over 170 board-certified dermatologists covering 34 states. It offers high-quality care by actual dermatologists while mimicking an in-office appointment, without all the driving and waiting.

You can start an online visit in one of two ways. You can sign up online at www.DermatologistOnCall.com. Or you can download the free mobile app from the App Store, Google Play, or the Amazon App Store.

You will select a preferred care provider, choose your pharmacy for any prescribed medications, and complete the medical forms. DermatologistOnCall accepts some insurance and reimbursement forms. You'll have to research your specific situation.

Next, you'll upload your "skin selfies" so the dermatologist can virtually examine your skin issues. You can expect a diagnosis and personal care treatment in 24 hours. DermatologistOnCall sends your prescription order to the pharmacy of your choice. It's fast, easy, and painless. The best part? As of the publication date of this book, the cost is only $59!

If your busy schedule is keeping you from getting proper treatment for your skin, then you may want to give DermatologistOnCall a try.

TWELVE

PRESCRIPTION MEDICATIONS FOR ACNE

Once you've had an appointment and discussed your skin with a dermatologist, he or she will prescribe your treatment plan. The following medications are the most common ones your dermatologist is likely to prescribe.

Oral Antibiotics

You may remember taking antibiotics such as tetracycline for years as a teenager. I know I did. These antibiotics don't work as well for adults; in fact, they hardly do, period. Over time, the organisms that antibiotics are supposed to kill adapt, making antibiotics less and less effective. Many countries report that 50% of P. acnes strains have developed resistance to antibiotics. According to the World Health Organization, resistance to antibiotics is an increasingly serious threat to global health.

Many dermatologists are concerned that the antibiotics

taken for acne can also create resistance among different types of bacteria in the body. The antibiotics clindamycin and doxycycline are often prescribed for acne, but they are also important treatments for some types of MRSA infections.

A dermatologist may prescribe antibiotics for a short time, typically no more than three to six months in order to jumpstart the clearing of your skin while you wait for other treatments to take effect, such as spironolactone or birth control pills. The most common antibiotics are clindamycin, doxycycline, erythromycin, and tetracycline.

Common side effects include:

- Dizziness
- Light-headedness
- Stomach aches
- Reduced effectiveness of birth control pills

Topical Antibiotics

The topical versions of the antibiotics listed above may also be prescribed. Like their oral counterparts, topical antibiotics may not work as well over time, as the bacteria on your skin develop resistance to them.

Many studies indicate that combining benzoyl peroxide with one of these antibiotics creates a more effective treatment. When combined, the antibiotics work faster, are more effective at reducing inflammation and the number of pimples, and antibiotic resistance is reduced. Apply topically once or twice a day after washing your face. You usually only need a small, pea-sized amount.

Dapsone

A 2016 study published in *The Journal of Drugs in Dermatology* found that a topical treatment of 5% dapsone gel (brand name Aczone) applied twice daily for 12 weeks reduced acne lesions between 50%-60%, with no side effects.

Dapsone is an antibiotic in the sulfone family of pharmaceuticals, and it's the relation to sulphur that provides its antibacterial benefits. Your dermatologist may prescribe Dapsone if other treatments don't work for you due to skin sensitivities, diminishing effectiveness, or side effects.

Spironolactone

Spironolactone is probably the number one treatment for hormonal acne in women, according to Dr. Tanzi. She is among hundreds of dermatologists around the country who highly recommend spironolactone.

Spironolactone was first used in 1957 to lower blood pressure and treat hypertension in patients with heart failure. It's a diuretic which causes people to urinate more, ridding the body of excess liquid while retaining the potassium the body needs to function. However, spironolactone also alters the way certain hormones are made and processed. The drug affects androgens, including testosterone.

Androgens in both men and women tell skin glands to

produce more oil, which clogs pores and leads to more acne. Spironolactone effectively blocks the receptors for these androgens, thereby reducing oil production. Even women with normal androgen levels can respond well to spironolactone.

Spironolactone has been used off-label for acne since the 1980s. While there are a few side effects, it is considered safe. One common side effect is irregular periods and spotting between periods. This usually normalizes within a few months as long as you take the medication regularly and at the same time each day. A rare side effect is too much potassium, which causes a condition called hyperkalemia. This can lead to heart arrhythmia. For this reason, dermatologists often have patients take periodic blood tests to monitor potassium levels.

However, in a September 2015 article published in *JAMA Dermatology*, Dr. Mostaghimi studied the records of 1000 healthy women taking spironolactone over a fifteen-year span. The rates of hyperkalemia were no higher than the general population, leading the researchers to conclude that screening is no longer necessary.

Spironolactone is typically given in initial doses of 50 to 100 mg twice daily, up to 200 mg a day. According to research, the expected reduction in acne is 33% to 85%. But results may vary. For me, it is 95%.

While men have positive results with spironolactone, the side effects for them are more severe, including decreased libido, impotence, and gynecomastia (enlarged breasts). For many men, the side effects are worse than the acne. For this reason, spironolactone is usually reserved for female patients.

Most common side effects include:

- Irregular periods
- Spotting in between periods
- Fatigue and drowsiness
- Nausea
- Breast pain, swelling
- Dizziness
- Headache

Birth Control Pills

"Women can try birth control pills to help their acne," says Dr. Debra Jaliman, a New York City board-certified dermatologist. The FDA has approved Estrostep, Ortho Tri-Cyclen, and Yaz for the treatment of acne. All three are combination pills, which means they contain estrogen and progesterone.

Birth control pills that contain both estrogen and progesterone reduce the amount of androgens in the body. The estrogen works by sponging up small amounts of testosterone. Lowered androgens means less oil, which means less acne. Progesterone-only pills won't work for acne, and neither will pills with low doses of estrogen. The ideal dose of estrogen seems to be about 30-35 micrograms.

Sometimes birth control pills are prescribed in conjunction with spironolactone. Estrogen therapy takes a few months to take effect, so be patient. Rare but serious side effects include leg blood clots. Be aware that some women experience severe moodiness and rapid mood swings.

Common side effects include:

- Headaches
- Breast tenderness
- Nausea
- Mood changes
- Lowered sex drive
- High blood pressure

Retinoids

Retinoids are derived from Vitamin A. Prescription-strength retinoids may be under a generic label or branded as Retin-A Micro, Renova, Avage, and Tazorac. "Retinoic acid is a gold standard that works on the comedone phase and through the inflammatory phase of acne," says Dr. Verallo-Rowell.

Our skin cells contain retinoid receptors which regulate skin cell functions. Retinoids improve skin texture and fade hyperpigmentation and sun spots because they promote the rapid turnover of new skin cells. This makes it less likely for pores to clog in the first place.

Retinoids also promote the retention of collagen. Collagen gives skin its firmness and elasticity. As we age (and expose ourselves to the sun), collagen breaks down, resulting in skin that wrinkles and sags.

Retinoids come in cream, gel, or liquid. Apply it once or twice a day 20-30 minutes after cleansing the skin. Note that waiting until your skin is completely dry is important to lessen dryness and irritation. When you first start treatment, you'll want to ease into it by applying it only once every couple of days.

Your skin will remain sensitive, so no peels, waxing, scrubs, or other harsh products.

You may also experience a purge, resulting in increased acne for a time while the pimples beneath your skin emerge. However, three different studies found no increase in acne during the initial weeks of treatment. If you do experience a purge, you should see improvement by the eight-week mark. Some individuals don't respond well to retinoids. For them, acne, irritation, and inflammation can worsen without ever getting better.

Dr. Verallo-Rowell recommends using retinoids but only under a doctor's supervision because of the intensity of side effects. And if you are pregnant or may be become pregnant, you need to avoid retinoids for now, as there is a small chance they can cause birth defects.

Dr. Verallo-Rowell cites a 2015 review and meta-analysis published in the *British Journal of Dermatology* that examined birth defects in 654 pregnant women who were exposed to topical retinoids and 1375 unexposed pregnant women. The researchers did not detect significant increases in rates of major congenital malformations, miscarriages, low birth weight, or prematurity. The majority of dermatologists still recommend avoiding retinoids during pregnancy, but if you are accidentally exposed, you don't need to be concerned.

Common side effects include:

- Excessive dryness
- Redness
- Itching

- Patchy, scaly skin
- Initial acne flare-up
- Blistering and stinging (rare)
- Skin discoloration (rare)

Isotretinoin

"Isotretinoin, also known as Accutane, can be very close to a cure," says Dr. Jaliman. She sees many patients cured of acne after one 20-week course. Dr. Cox also finds Accutane as the most consistently effective treatment for persistent acne, with high patient satisfaction. Several studies show a six-month course of isotretinoin clears up to 95% of patients. For 85% of patients, the improvement can last for several years, according to the American Academy of Dermatology.

Isotretinoin is in a class of medications known as retinoids, derived from vitamin A. It works by both reducing the size of the skin's oil glands and reducing the amount of oil the glands produce. It also slows how quickly the skin produces skin cells inside each pore, so pores become less clogged. The dosage ranges from 0.5 to 1.0 mg/kg of body weight per day. Patients who receive a cumulative dose (over 18 to 20 weeks) of 100-120 mg/kg see the best results. Researchers have experimented with lowering the dosage for a longer period of time, achieving similar results without as many side effects.

Isotretinoin can be a life-changer. It is also a serious medication. It is an internal retinoid which needs to be monitored with blood tests. It can take months to be effective, and acne may worsen before it gets better. Side effects are very common (up to 80% of patients) and can be frustrating to deal with. More serious side effects include birth defects and gastrointestinal disorders such as Crohn's disease.

Common side effects include:

- Sun sensitivity
- Dry, cracked lips
- Nosebleeds
- Peeling skin
- Unusual hair growth or loss
- Bleeding or swollen gums
- Headache
- Dry skin and eyes
- Muscle aches
- Depression

Case Study

Ashleigh DePalma has struggled with acne for much of her 29 years. She's used just about everything, from benzoyl peroxide, retinoids, chemical peels, antibiotics, and hormonal treatments. Nothing worked for her. After years of frustration, she finally decided isotretinoin was worth the risk.

She's now on a high dose of isotretinoin. Her side effects include dry lips, dry eyes, dry skin, eczema, and a dry nose. Her skin is also more sensitive. But it's working for her. Her skin is already much clearer, and she's hopeful the results will be permanent.

So far, she hasn't experienced any of the more serious side effects. "It's a drug that can cause a lot of side effects, but I wish I would have tried it sooner and saved myself a lot of embarrassment and heartache," DePalma says.

THIRTEEN

NATURAL ACNE REMEDIES

The problem with natural remedies is that there is very little empirical research on their effectiveness. Anecdotal stories and reviews populate the internet, but hard evidence is elusive. I recommend studying the reviews on sites like Acne.org and Makeupalley.com to decide for yourself which methods you might like to try.

I also recommend talking to your doctor before trying anything new. "Natural products do not necessarily equate with safe," warns Dr. Verallo-Rowell. "Mangoes are natural, so are strawberries and peanuts. Yet they are often very allergenic." Just because something is natural doesn't mean it is safe, or that you can't overdose on good-for-you vitamins and minerals.

I've included the most popular natural remedies in this chapter.

Tea Tree Oil

There are a few natural treatments that have received some attention from the scientific community. Certain essential oils have been the subject of several studies, most notably tea tree oil. Dr. Tanzi and Dr. Jaliman both recommend 5% tea tree oil for its antibacterial, acne-killing properties.

This essential oil is extracted from the leaves of a tree native to Australia. Back in 1990, researchers tested tea tree oil against 5% benzoyl peroxide. While the tea tree oil took a little longer to work, it was just as effective as benzoyl peroxide, sans the drying, irritating side effects.

Tea tree oil is too strong undiluted. Mix 5-10 drops in ¼ cup water, or one teaspoon of oil to nine teaspoons of water, then apply to your face with a cotton ball. Repeat up to 2x per day.

Some people may be allergic to this essential oil. So make sure to test a small area first. Tea tree oil should never be taken orally, as it can cause a serious toxic reaction that can lead to coma.

Jojoba Oil

Jojoba oil (pronounced hohoba) won't clear acne, but it is an excellent soothing, calming moisturizer. It can also be used as a face wash. Contrary to popular opinion, this type of oil won't make your skin oilier. It restores balance and needed moisture to your skin. If jojoba oil feels too "oily" on your skin, you can mix it with pure aloe before applying it to your face. You only need a few drops.

Calming oils like jojoba are also great to use after a peel to really soothe your skin. It can also be used on your hair as a frizz smoother and leave-in conditioner. Remember, a little goes a long way! Too much oil in your hair can be extremely difficult to wash out. As a frizz smoother, add one or two drops, rub into your palms, and run your fingers through damp or dry hair.

Other Essential oils

Several essential oils have antibacterial properties that can help reduce acne. A 2010 study published in *Molecules Journal* found that cinnamon, thyme, and rose essential oils showed the best antibacterial effects. But thyme and cinnamon can be too harsh. Rose essential oil is both antibacterial and anti-inflammatory, so it can calm redness and irritation.

Green Tea

Green tea contains antimicrobial and antioxidant compounds which help acne when used as a tea and topically. A 2010 study in *Journal of Drugs in Dermatology* found green tea effective in combating acne and rosacea. And a 2012 review of over 20 studies in *SKINmed: A Journal of Dermatology for Clinicians* found green tea was effective both topically and orally.

To use orally, drink two to five cups a day. To use topically, try laying a freshly used bag over the affected area for five minutes. You can also dip a washcloth in chilled green tea, wring it out, and then press gently to the affected area for 1-2 minutes. Repeat 4-5 times. This method is great for calming redness and inflammation.

Zinc

Dr. Jaliman recommends adding a zinc supplement to your acne regimen. Zinc is a trace element which is essential to all forms of life. It plays a critical role in cell growth and cell replication. It also plays a key role in the proper function of insulin, which makes it doubly important for clear skin.

Zinc is also one of the most studied natural treatments for acne. It is naturally anti-inflammatory and antibacterial. It is also an antioxidant. Zinc helps the pores of the skin stay open by reducing keratin, a tough protein that binds skin cells together, clogging pores. Zinc is also a mild DHT blocker, meaning it reduces the effect hormones have on the skin. Now, if you are already getting adequate amounts of zinc, taking more is unlikely to do much for your acne.

However, according to the World Health Organization, up to 31.7% of the world's population is zinc-deficient. A 2014 study in *Biomed Research International* found a correlation between serum zinc levels in the blood and the severity and type of acne the study subjects suffered from. Research shows that, on average, people with acne have 24% lower zinc levels than people without acne.

If you are one of the one-in-three people without enough zinc, a supplement could improve your acne—and by a significant amount. In a large 2001 study in *Dermatology*, subjects who took 30 mg of zinc a day over twelve weeks saw an overall decrease in the number of pimples by nearly 50%.

A therapeutic dose is about 30 mg per day. Studies show that zinc picolinate has the best bioavailability, i.e., the body can utilize it the best.

Of course, talk to your doctor before implementing any new plan, especially if you are already taking other medications. Too much zinc may cause nausea, vomiting, diarrhea, and kidney and stomach damage. Take zinc during or after a meal to avoid an upset stomach.

Coconut Oil

Dr. Verallo-Rowell recommends using coconut oil not just for cooking but as a moisturizer and/or makeup remover. Coconut oil is one of the richest sources of lauric acid, which is anti-fungal, antibacterial, and anti-inflammatory. A 2009 study published in *Biomaterials* proved that lauric acid was an excellent inhibitor of the bacteria *P. acnes*. It also has plenty of vitamin E and healthy fats to lubricate and plump the skin.

Like other medications, both natural and manmade, breakouts are part of the detoxification process as the deeper grime, pollution, and inflammation come to the surface.

Make sure the coconut oil you use is virgin or extra virgin and organic. Your typical store-bought coconut oil contains added ingredients which could aggravate your acne.

To use, massage a teaspoon of coconut oil into clean skin for a few minutes. Rinse with water and a gentle cleanser. To use as a makeup remover, massage into your skin with water. Use cotton pads or a soft washcloth to wipe away makeup. You can finish up with a cotton ball of apple cider vinegar mixed with water as a gentle toner.

Aloe

You usually use aloe for sunburn to relieve redness and burning. But aloe also promotes healing, fights infections, and reduces scarring. Scientists believe it is the anti-inflammatory compounds aloin and aloesin which make aloe so effective. However, it must be pure aloe—with no added ingredients—to work properly. You can scrape the gel directly from the plant or buy it pure from health food stores. To use, massage it into your skin at night before bed or apply to affected pimples.

Apple Cider Vinegar

This vinegar contains acetic acids which are antibacterial, antifungal, and naturally exfoliate and reduce red marks. People use apple cider vinegar for almost everything, from diabetes and heart issues to high cholesterol and weight loss.

Make sure the vinegar contains the "mother", i.e. strands of proteins, friendly bacteria, and enzymes that make the liquid murky but effective. The typical stuff you grab at the grocery store won't cut it. Try Bragg's organic, unfiltered brand. And always shake well before use.

To use, mix equal parts vinegar and water and apply to skin with a cotton ball. If that's too strong, you can dilute 2-3 teaspoons with ¼ cup water. You can also take 1 tbsp. a day orally.

Omega-3 fatty acids

We've already talked about the benefits of Omega-3s as an anti-inflammatory acne fighter in chapter seven. Aim for 2000 mg a day in a fish oil supplement (wild-caught salmon is the purest source). Increase your flaxseed and walnut intake. Try one tablespoon of flaxseed on top of steel cut oatmeal and a handful of walnuts a day. Look for a high-quality supplement with plenty of DHA and EPA.

Raw Honey

Raw, unfiltered honey contains antiseptic qualities, which helps it fight the *P. acnes* bacteria and heal scars from cystic acne. Fans claim Manuka honey heals scars the fastest. Honey is also a great moisturizer that won't clog your pores.

Use raw, unfiltered honey (buy at Amazon or health food stores) as a mask 1x to 3x a week. Apply one teaspoon to your face. Leave on for 10 to 15 minutes and rinse.

Baking Soda Mask

Baking soda, or sodium bicarbonate, contains some antiseptic and anti-inflammatory properties. It helps eliminate breakouts and reduces redness and inflammation. Baking soda's round, hard particles make it an excellent mild exfoliator to help remove dead skin cells.

To use, mix a teaspoon of baking soda with warm water until it forms a paste. You can also mix a teaspoon of baking soda with a teaspoon of lemon juice. Apply the paste to your skin for 3-5 minutes. You can gradually increase the time.

Use once a week. Make sure you do a spot test to ensure it won't irritate your skin.

Bentonite Clay Mask

Bentonite clay, or Montmorillonite, is a natural, quarry-mined clay that includes minerals such as iron, sodium, calcium, potassium and magnesium. It is highly absorbent, and when it is mixed with a liquid, it develops a mild electrical charge that helps it to draw toxins, heavy metals and other impurities out of the pores. Its astringent properties work to shrink enlarged pores and soften skin.

Clean your face with water first. Mix a few teaspoons of clay (it comes in powder form) with an equal amount of water. You can add a few drops of tea tree oil or apple cider vinegar. Do not use a metal spoon or bowl, because metals from the spoon will leach into the clay, diminishing its effectiveness.

Leave the mask on for 20 to 30 minutes. You'll feel your skin tightening as it dries. Rinse off the mask with water.

Spot Treatments

Sometimes you need to deflate a pimple fast or lessen redness for a big event or meeting. Here are the best spot treatments to help reduce inflammation overnight. Several methods already mentioned include a green tea bag compress, tea tree oil (diluted), and products containing sulfur.

Lemon: Lemons are high in vitamin C and will help dry out the pimple. Squeeze lemon juice on a cotton ball and press it against the pimple for two minutes. It's drying so it works to get rid of excess oils and reduce the overall appearance pretty quickly.

Ice: Ice can minimize swelling and alleviate pain. Wrap an ice cube in a paper towel and press it to the affected blemish. You can also freeze green tea in ice cube form for a double dose of redness-reducing power.

Aspirin: Aspirin contains a compound very similar to salicylic acid. It reduces inflammation and redness and clears out pores. Wash your face with warm water. For a small area, crush an uncoated aspirin tablet and mix it with a few drops of distilled (bottled) water to form a paste. Apply it to the area and leave it on for several minutes.

To use as a mask, crush 7-8 uncoated aspirin tablets with a few drops of water and one teaspoon of organic honey. You can sub jojoba oil for the honey if you're dealing with dryness. Apply to your face and leave on for 7-15 minutes.

FOURTEEN

ALL ABOUT CHEMICAL PEELS

CHEMICAL PEELS ARE an integral part of my acne arsenal—and they should be part of yours, as well. Peels reach deeper layers of the skin than do traditional topical products. Chemical peels clear out pores, remove the top layer of skin for a bright healthy glow, kill bacteria to reduce acne, and minimize fine lines and wrinkles. Deeper chemical peels can lighten red marks and fade scarring.

Where to Buy Chemical Peels

Most of us don't have the time or the funds to drop $100 or more at the spa every few weeks for professional chemical peels. But there is an amazing company called Makeup Artist's Choice (www.muac.com) that sells professional, pharmaceutical grade chemical peels to consumers to use at home. This is not Amazon or eBay, where you can't be sure what you might get. Be very careful where you source a product like a chemical peel. Never mess around when you're putting acid on your face!

But Makeup Artist's Choice is for real. They use FDA-registered laboratory facilities and produce top quality, medical grade peels. They have a ton of great reviews, and they've been in business for years. You can buy from them with confidence. I have no association with MUAC whatsoever, other than the fact that their chemical peels helped save my skin.

Chemical Peels 101

Chemical peels are broadly defined by their depth. They are categorized as superficial, medium, and deep. Superficial peels don't reach the skin below the epidermis, the top layer of skin. Medium peels may reach the next layer of the skin, the dermis. Deep peels reach the deeper layers of the dermis. Tread cautiously here. If you try a deep chemical peel, you can expect severe redness, flaking, and oozing skin for anywhere from one to four weeks as your skin repairs itself.

Dr. Trakimas recommends fruit-acid-based chemical peels like glycolic acid peels, beta hydroxy peels, and/or lactic acid peels—all of which can treat acne and help fade red marks.

Alpha Hydroxy Acids

Alpha hydroxy acids (or AHAs) are derived from milk and fruit sugars. They've been popular for thousands of years because of their ability to penetrate the skin. Cleopatra is said to have bathed in sour milk (lactic acid) to improve her complexion.

Alpha hydroxy acids work mainly as an exfoliator. They slough off dead skin cells, making room for the regrowth of new skin. Alpha hydroxy acids may even stimulate the production of collagen and elastin. Low level AHAs are often added to moisturizers, cleansers, and toners.

There are five types of AHAs:

- glycolic acid – sugar cane
- lactic acid – milk
- malic acid – apples and pears
- citric acid – oranges and lemons
- tartaric acid – grapes

Beta Hydroxy Acid

There is only one beta-hydroxy acid (BHA): salicylic acid. The main difference between the two is that BHA is oil-soluble. AHAs are water-soluble. Beta hydroxy acid is better able to penetrate into the oily pore and really exfoliate those trapped dead skin cells. This makes salicylic acid excellent for oily skin, blackheads, and whiteheads.

How to Peel

I've collated a list of the best peels for acne-prone skin. Peels come in different strengths. *Always* start with the lowest strength and the shortest amount of time. Follow instructions and slowly work your way up with longer times and increased strengths.

Peels can damage your skin if you leave them on for too long or start with a peel that's too strong. Before using any peel, test a small area of your skin first to make sure you aren't allergic. Remember, these are the professional-strength peels that clinicians and dermatologists use themselves. When used properly, peels can do wonders for your skin. If used improperly, they can cause scarring and other damage.

Generally, you will do a peel once a week for four to six weeks. Lower strength peels can be used once a week indefinitely. You can work your way up to strong enough peels where the top layer of your skin will actually peel off over several days. Because I can't take time off of work, I typically don't use stronger peels. A low-strength salicylic or lactic acid peel once a week keeps pores tight and clear and your skin bright and free of excess oil.

Remember, irritating your acne can backfire. Harsh peels can sometimes make things worse. Don't be so gung-ho to improve your skin that you make things worse in the process. Gentle peels can be extremely effective if you are patient and give them some time to do their work.

Before doing any peel, make sure you follow all instructions to a T, including:

- Don't scrub skin for 24 hours before using a peel.
- Make sure you stop harsh acne products 24 hours before AND after using a peel.
- If you are allergic to aspirin, peels aren't for you.

- Don't apply a chemical peel to inflamed skin.

Lactic Acid

This is the best peel for beginners and those with sensitive skin, hands down. I still use this peel weekly with excellent results.

Lactic acid is a non-irritating exfoliator. It softens fine lines and deep-cleans pores. It stimulates natural collagen production and is great for brightening all skin types, including mature skin. What's particularly nice is that the skin doesn't really flake—it sloughs off oil and skin debris without being noticeable.

Caution: If you have a milk allergy, avoid this peel. Lactic acid peels come in strengths beginning at 40% and go up to 65%.

Salicylic Acid Peels

Salicylic acid peels promote the removal of dead skin cells from the top layers of skin. The salicylic acid peel also has antibacterial properties that help with active acne. Pores will look smaller and tighter, and your skin will feel and look smooth and bright. This peel is great for blackheads.

Salicylic peels are gentle and have no down time (i.e., your skin is so red or peeling so badly you don't want to show your face to the world). They start at 15% and go up to 30%.

Glycolic Acid Peels

Glycolic acid peels also remove dead, dull cells on the top layer of skin. It refines and smooths skin texture and unclogs pores. Your skin is then better able to absorb moisture. Some people experience irritation with glycolic acid. It made me break out for weeks. When I switched to salicylic and lactic acid, the breakouts stopped.

Remember though, sometimes the breakout is just a purge. At the beginning of treatment, your pores are congested and blocked with dirt, oil, and bacteria. The sebum already present under the surface will emerge as blemishes. The acid is cleaning the pores much more quickly than regular products. Your skin should start improving within three to four weeks.

This peel also has no downtime. Strengths start at 30% and go up to 70%.

Jessner's Peel

This is a popular medium-depth chemical peel that works well for back and chest acne and cystic acne. It's also great for sun-damaged skin. It is made up of lactic acid, salicylic acid, and resorcinol, all of which help improve acne. The Jessner's peel works by loosening acne that's deep in the skin. It tightens large pores and reduces acne scarring.

You will have peeling with a Jessner's peel. Two to five coats are applied until your skin "frosts". Frosting occurs when your skin turns white during a peel. Once your skin starts to frost, it is time to rinse. It will sting! Your skin will be tight, dry, and sensitive afterward. The peeling will start within several days and continue for about a week. When the old skin peels away, newer, fresher skin is revealed.

This peel can be repeated once a month, but it is so strong that many people see great results with one peel. Avoid this peel if you are pregnant or have been on Accutane in the last six months.

TCA Peel

A trichloroacetic acid (TCA) peel is the big gun of the chemical peel world. TCA is the same main ingredient used in the wildly popular Obagi Blue Peel. This peel is excellent at softening deeper wrinkles, rapidly fading red marks, and at reducing acne scars more dramatically than lighter peels.

Because these peels are so strong, be very careful if you choose to use this at home. I recommend saving deep peels like TCA peels for the experts. That being said, many people have done them successfully at home with good results.

"I did an 18% double layer and my progress was amazing," says Neal Moore of South Bend, Indiana. "My acne scars have greatly diminished and my skin is smoother. My friend and sister both deal with hyperpigmentation, and they both have seen significant fading of their spots."

There will be noticeable peeling and you will need to take some time off. Your skin will look severely sunburned. Expect your skin to heal within five to seven days. The skin will turn reddish brown and crusty in two to three days, like the patient pictured below.

Don't be alarmed. This is a normal part of the process. Over the next few days, your brown, crusty skin will flake and peel, slowly revealing the bright, healthy skin underneath.

Make sure you follow the directions very carefully. Possible complications like scarring and hyperpigmentation become more serious with stronger peels.

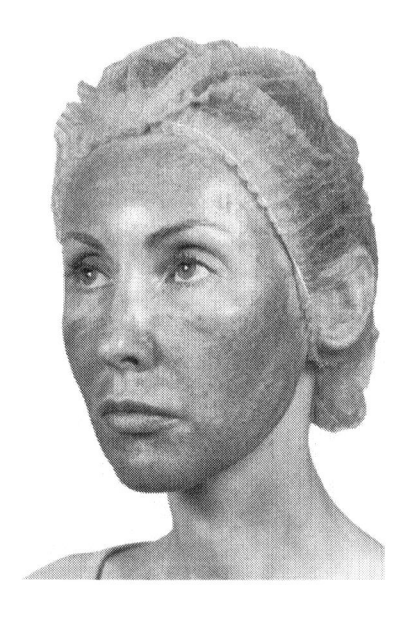

Strengths vary from 12.5% to 24%. At percentages of 15% and higher, you may get the results you want after a single peel. According to MUAC:

- 12.5% is a light peel.
- 15% is a light-medium peel.
- 18% is a medium peel.
- 21% is a medium-strong peel. It should be used ONLY by clients who have tolerated the 18% well.

- 24% is a strong peel.

Make sure you start low and work your way up. The 21% and 24% peels are deeper peels. Do not use the 18% peel unless you've already tried the 15%.

These peels typically cost several hundred dollars per peel at a doctor's office. Avoid this peel if you have used Accutane within the last 24 months. People with darker skin tones shouldn't go above 15%.

At a spa or plastic surgeon's office, light peels like glycolic acid peels range from $75 to $150 per session. Deeper peels like a TCA peel range from $300 to $1000 a session.

Chemical Peel risks/side effects

The deeper the peel, the higher the chance of side effects.

- Redness, peeling, crusting (part of healing process)
- Scarring (rare)
- Hyperpigmentation (likelier with darker complexions)

Chemical peels are excellent at tightening pores and fading hyperpigmentation, which I'll talk about more in the next chapter.

FIFTEEN

HYPERPIGMENTATION AND SCARRING

Sometimes the red marks and scars left behind by the ravages of acne can be worse than the pimples themselves. "Long after the active acne, people can still be unhappy about their skin," says Dr. Verallo-Rowell. Even though it is incredibly hard to resist, don't pop your pimples. Acne scarring and pitting is hard to diminish. So don't scar yourself in the first place.

According to the American Society for Dermatologic Surgery, acne scars result when the acne-inflamed pore swells and causes a rupture in the follicle wall. When there is a deep break in the pore wall, the body attempts to repair the large lesions by creating new collagen fibers. But these repairs, like other types of scars, are not smooth and flawless.

"Serious scars can range from 'rolling hills' to 'icepick' to 'boxcar,'" explains Dr. Verallo-Rowell. Scars are difficult to treat because they affect the deep layers of the skin.

However, "Dermatologists offer multiple options that provide excellent results when it comes to the treatment of scarring," says Dr. Jeremy Brauer, a dermatologic surgeon, a clinician assistant professor at NYU Langone Medical Center, and the Director of Clinical Research at the Laser and Skin Surgery Center of New York. "With that being said, not all scarring is amenable to treatment." It's important to enter treatment with realistic expectations. Your scars may never completely fade away, but they can be softened and diminished.

Chemical Peels

Chemical peels are excellent at completely fading hyperpigmentation and reducing scarring. Chapter 14 contains more detailed information on chemical peels. The great thing about peels is that you can do them at home, cheaply—not so with lasers.

Laser Resurfacing

Lasers can work well for moderate to severe cases if you have the money to spend on them. Lasers resurface the skin by vaporizing the top layers of skin tissue to promote the body's wound-healing response, which stimulates collagen production.

There are two major types of laser treatments, ablative and non-ablative. Ablative treatments use very high temperatures to destroy the epidermis and dermis layers of the skin. While they can be very effective, the treatment comes with significant side effects and several weeks of recovery.

Nonablative treatments are gentler, with fewer side effects and less downtime. The results are not as dramatic, and several treatments are required. For scarring, Dr. Brauer recommends both ablative and nonablative fraxel lasers, as does Dr. Cox.

A fraxel laser uses "fractional photothermolysis", a technology which utilizes thousands of microscopic laser columns which treat a fraction of the skin at a time. The laser stimulates the production of smoother, healthier skin to replace the damaged, scarred tissue.

A 2016 study in the journal *Lasers in Medical Science* studied acne-scar patients treated over three monthly sessions with a fractional CO_2 laser. At the sixth-month follow-up, 95% of patients reported moderate to excellent healing of scars. Another 2014 study in *Journal of Cutaneous and Aesthetic Surgery* found that 43% of patients had excellent results, 25% had good results, and about 32% had a poor response.

This varied effectiveness rate is reflected by the mixed experiences on review sites like Acne.org. Proceed with caution. Make sure you use an experienced doctor, and make sure you have realistic expectations.

Laser Treatment

Even though a scalpel is not involved, laser resurfacing is generally considered surgery by plastic surgeons due to the severity of the wounds lasers cause and the anesthesia required. Recovery time varies depending on the type of laser. For a CO_2 laser, recovery time can be two weeks. For the fraxel laser, recovery may be only a few days.

Costs vary wildly. Do your research. Visit a few different doctors to compare quotes. But expect laser treatment to be expensive. "A full face treatment can range from hundreds to thousands of dollars depending upon what device is used," says Dr. Brauer. According to the American Society of Plastic Surgeons, the average fees for laser resurfacing are about $2500.

It will take several sessions to see improvement. Sessions are usually a month apart. The best results are usually obtained with a combination of procedures.

Side effects/risks include:

- Temporary redness, swelling, and bruising
- Permanently lightened or darkened skin
- Hyperpigmentation of laser-treated areas
- Burns
- Additional scarring
- Bacterial infection

What to Look for in a Doctor

"It is very important that a patient select a board-certified dermatologist with sufficient and appropriate training with the devices they recommend," says Dr. Brauer. Look for a doctor with extensive experience and years of training in the laser you're considering.

Be honest with your doctor about your expectations, your available down time, how quickly you want to achieve results, and your pain tolerance level. The answers to these questions will help determine the best treatment choice for you. Don't be afraid to ask your doctor plenty of questions. You want to be comfortable with your treatment decisions. Ask for references.

Microdermabrasion

Microdermabrasion is an alternative to chemical peels. The procedure uses a wand to blast your face with aluminum oxide or salt crystal microparticles to rub off the top layer of skin, then vacuum up the particles and dead skin cells.

Microdermabrasion removes the outer layer of the epidermis and deeply exfoliates the skin. Microdermabrasion is painless, but it is also not as effective as some other treatments. And it doesn't treat deep scars, such as ice pick or boxcar scars. It can improve rough skin texture, fine wrinkles, and hyperpigmentation. Results are similar to a light chemical peel, with no anesthesia and no downtime. Side effects are minimal.

Each treatment takes 30-45 minutes and consists of four to eight treatments conducted two to four weeks apart. Costs are usually between $150 to $350 per session.

SIXTEEN

YOUR CLEAR SKIN ACTION PLAN

"Acne can be managed," says Waller. She compares it to weight loss. "If you return to what got you overweight to begin with, then the weight returns. It's the same with acne." Small changes over time will make a large impact. Build new habits, and soon the changes in your routine will seem natural. Incorporate the following guidelines into your daily routine to change your skin for good. You can start as soon as today.

Wash What Touches Your Face

Regularly wash your towels, sheets, pillowcases, washcloths, makeup brushes, hats, and anything else that touches your face—including your hands. Actually, touch your face with your hands as little as possible.

Use Gentle Cleansers

The American Academy of Dermatology recommends throwing away your astringents, toners, and harsh cleansers. "They strip the skin's natural moisture barrier, which leaves it vulnerable to bacteria," says Waller. Instead, wash your face twice a day, using a gentle, sensitive-skin cleanser such as Aveeno Ultra Calming Face Wash or natural oils like jojoba or coconut oil. Add a drop to your hands, massage into your face, then rinse.

Gordon gave up her harsh cleansers. They only dried her out, which stimulated excess oil production. She started using water only, and it worked for her. "Good old H$_2$O is still my favorite cleanser today!"

Avoid Irritation

Gentleness is key. Don't scrub your face. Avoid abrasive products like acne scrubs, rough washcloths, etc. Whatever you do, don't pick at your skin. This just irritates your acne and can make inflammation worse.

Apply Your Acne Treatment

Whether you're using benzoyl peroxide or a prescription antibiotic, apply it sparingly after your clean skin is dry. In the evening, once your skin is dry after washing your face, apply a retinoid or AHA treatment.

Wear Sunscreen

While sunscreen doesn't actually combat acne, it does prevent sun damage. While a tan can make you look great for a few days, sun damage causes skin imbalance and slows down your skin's proper functions. It exacerbates acne by damaging and irritating the top layers of your skin.

"Sun protection, sun protection, sun protection," says Dr. Brauer. It's that important. "Appropriate use of broad spectrum UVA/UVB sunscreen is critical for patients suffering from acne and acne scarring."

Moisturize Effectively

Look for an oil-free, water-based moisturizer and use it daily. If you have sensitive skin, find one without fragrance. You can also use a small amount of calming, hydrating essential oils.

Peel Once a Week

Apply a light chemical peel once a week to exfoliate the top layer of skin, fight acne bacteria, and lessen red marks over time.

Dump Your Products in the Trash

Dr. Verallo-Rowell recommends using as few products as possible. Too many harsh products can have the opposite effect of what you're going for. Use the cosDNA website and the Acne-Causing Ingredients List at the end of this book to comb through the ingredients of every product that touches your face.

Get rid of anything with more than one or two ingredients rated a three or higher in the first eight ingredients.

Replace Your Makeup

Search out gentle, non-irritating, and non-clogging products to use in your foundation, concealers, powder, blush, etc. Look for sheer, water-based products and use sparingly. Don't exercise while wearing makeup if you can avoid it!

Get Your Vitamin D

A fifteen-minute walk outside every day can help combat acne. Sunlight enables your body to produce Vitamin D, which helps fight inflammation.

Guzzle Up

"I always recommend drinking enough water each day so that your body and skin remain hydrated," says Dr. Bank. Water won't actually prevent acne, but it will help your skin stay moisturized. Hydration is necessary for detoxification, which helps flush out toxins and balance your hormones. Dehydrated skin produces more sebum to overcompensate for the needed lubrication. And we know where that cycle leads.

How much is enough? Six to eight glasses a day to start with. Bring water bottles with you to work. Drink one to two glasses at every meal.

Feed Your Skin

Throughout the day, choose high antioxidant, low glycemic foods to promote healthy skin from the inside out. Fight inflammation and oxidative stress by eating naturally colorful foods that are full of vitamins and minerals. Drink a few cups of green tea a day.

"The most important things that you can do for your complexion is to eat a diet that's rich in antioxidants and to apply excellent products recommended by your dermatologist," says Dr. Trakimas.

Avoid Your Trigger Foods

Conduct a twelve-week elimination diet to discover which foods are your particular trigger foods. Stay as close to a 100% clean diet as you can, but understand that you can have an occasional cheat meal and still see good results.

After you've discovered your trigger foods, whether that's dairy, just milk, refined sugar, processed carbs, or all of the above, cut them 90-100% out of your diet. Many people can still have a couple of servings of dairy or dessert a week and maintain their clear skin. Remember, you don't have to be perfect to be successful!

Supplement Sparingly

With your doctor's approval, take a high-quality omega-3 supplement, aiming for 2000-3000 mg a day to fight inflammation. Also with your doctor's approval, you can try a 30-mg zinc supplement.

Visit A Dermatologist

If your acne is moderate to severe or you suspect hormonal acne, schedule an appointment to see a dermatologist. He or she may prescribe antibiotics, hormone therapy like spironolactone, and/or retinoid treatment. Follow your doctor's instructions and give any new medication a few months to work.

Give It Time

Remember, take things one step at a time and realize it may take several months to see real results. Acne starts deep inside, and it takes time to clear out and detoxify your system. "Don't get overwhelmed," Waller recommends. "Make a plan and stick to it, and your skin will reflect those changes."

Love Yourself

This is the most important step of all. Love yourself, regardless of what your skin looks like. "Don't let acne rule your life or it will ruin your life," Gordon says. She's right. If you keep telling yourself you can't really live until your skin is clear, you are missing out on some wonderful memories and life experiences.

Get out there and enjoy your life. The reality is that the people who are most worth having in your life are the ones who will love and support you for who you are, not for what your skin looks like. "Enjoy friends and be your own best friend as well," suggests Dr. Verallo-Rowell.

Learn to love yourself, acne scars and all. Of course you want clear, healthy skin. But clear skin isn't going to solve all your problems. It won't bring you happiness. That has to come from within.

SEVENTEEN

THOUGHTS FROM THE OTHER SIDE

REMEMBER TO CHECK out the following chapters for even more great resources: Chapter 18: Websites and Product Recommendations; Chapter 19: Acne-Causing Ingredients List; and Chapter 20: Your Clear Skin Diet Plan.

I hope you found the information in this book valuable. Adult acne is a physical and emotional burden no one should have to bear. Remember to be patient, to realize that what worked for someone else won't necessarily work for you, and that your clear skin journey is just that—a journey.

You will find what works best for you, but it may take some time. Give your new lifestyle a few months to work its magic.

And when it does, I want to hear about it. Let me know what in this book worked for you and what didn't. And if something completely different helped you, I'd love to know that, too, so I can include it in the next edition of *Real Solutions for Adult Acne*.

If you found this book useful, please don't forget to add a quick review on Amazon. Even just a two-word "Liked It" really helps add visibility and support so that other people can find and enjoy this book as well.

Want to know when my next book is available? Sign up for my new release email alerts! You will get special access to deep discounts and sales.

Visit my author page at Facebook.com/KylaStoneBooks or Facebook.com/AdultAcne and click on the email signup link!

EIGHTEEN

WEBSITE AND PRODUCT RECOMMENDATIONS

These are the websites and products I and many other adult acne sufferers recommend.

Always check with your doctor before starting new supplements or medications.

Websites

www.Acne.org
www.MakeupArtistsChoice.com
www.PaulasChoice.com
www.MakeupAlley.com
www.CosDNA.com
www.DermatologistOnCall.com

Recommended Products

Moisturizer
100% Pure & Natural Golden Jojoba Oil (Unrefined)
Calamine Lotion
CeraVe Moisturizing Lotion
Grandma Minnie's Oil's Well Nurturing Do-It-Oil

Sunscreen
Aveeno Ultra-Calming Daily Moisturizer SPF 15
Neutrogena Clear Face Sunblock Lotion, SPF 30

Cleanser
Purpose Gentle Cleansing Wash
Aveeno Ultra Calming Foaming Cleanser

Coconut Oil
Carrington Farms Extra Virgin Organic Coconut Oil
VMV Hypoallergenics Know-It-Oil, 100% USDA-certified organic cold-pressed virgin coconut oil

Bentonite Clay Mask
Aztec Secret Indian Healing Clay Deep Pore Cleansing

Omega-3 Supplement
Viva Labs Ultra Strength Omega-3 Fish Oil, 2200 mg

OmegaVia Fish Oil, 1105 mg
NutriGold Triple Strength Omega-3 Fish Oil, 1250 mg

Zinc Picolinate Supplement
    Garden of Life Vitamin Code Zinc, 30 mg
    NOW Foods Zinc Picolinate, 50 mg
    Solgar Zinc Picolinate Tablets, 22 mg

Probiotics
    Healthy Origins Probiotic 30 Billion CFU's Shelf Stable
    Renew Life Ultimate Flora Probiotic 50 Billion
    Sedona Labs Iflora Multi-Probiotic Formula

Tea Tree Oil
    Thursday Plantation 100% Pure Tea Tree Oil

Raw Manuka Honey
    Kiva Certified UMF 15+ Raw Manuka Honey
    Wild Cape UMF 10+ Manuka Honey
    Trader Joe's Manuka Honey 10+

Vinegar Apple Cider with mother
    Bragg Organic Raw Apple Cider Vinegar

Green Tea
Stash Tea Premium Green Tea, Tea Bags in Foil
KENKO Matcha Green Tea Powder Organic

Chemical peels
Anything from Makeup Artist's Choice

NINETEEN

ACNE-CAUSING INGREDIENTS LIST

THE FOLLOWING LIST includes common ingredients in cosmetics, powders, lotions, concealers, creams, etc. that can cause acne. Don't expect to find products completely free of these ingredients, and don't be surprised when you find some known acnegenic ingredients included in a supposedly anti-acne product on the shelves of a beauty store or advertised on television.

You should also know that this list is primarily based on a study conducted in 2005 using rabbit ear assays. It was not conducted on human skin. "Rabbit ear assay continues to be used for rating comedogenicity of cosmetics despite conflicting results versus human skin assay," explains Dr. Verallo-Rowell. In a soon-to-be-published study conducted by Dr. Verallo-Rowell, the team of researchers tested eight different oils on human skin and found that out of avocado, castor, extra virgin olive oil, grapeseed, safflower, sunflower, almond oil, and virgin coconut oil, only almond oil caused acne. All that to say, study this list with a grain of salt.

Acetylated Lanolin
> 4

Acetylated Lanolin Alcohol
> 4

Algae Extract
> 5

Algin
> 4

Butyl Stearate
> 3

Carrageenan
> 5

Cetearyl Alcohol + Ceteareth 20
> 4

Cetyl Acetate
> 4

Cocoa Butter
> 4

Colloidal Sulfur
> 3

Cotton Awws Oil
> 3

Cottonseed Oil
> 3

Crisco
3
D & C Red #17
3
D & C Red #21
3
D & C Red #3
3
D & C Red #30
3
D & C Red #36
3
Decyl Oleate
3
Dioctyl Succinate
3
Disodium Oleamido PEG 2-Sulfosuccinate
4
Ethoxylated Lanolin
3
Ethylhexyl Palmitate
4
Glyceryl Stearate SE
3
Glyceryl-3-Diisostearate
4
Hexadecyl Alcohol
5

Hydrogenated Vegetable Oil

3

Isocetyl Alcohol

4

Isocetyl Stearate

5

Isodecyl Oleate

4

Isopropyl Isostearate

5

Isopropyl Linolate

5

Isopropyl Myristate

5

Isopropyl Palmitate

4

Isostearyl Isostearate

4

Isostearyl Neopentanoate

3

Laureth 23

3

Laureth 4

5

Lauric Acid

4

Mink Oil

3

Myristic Acid
3
Myristyl Lactate
4
Myristyl Myristate
5
Octyl Palmitate
4
Octyl Stearate
5
Oleth-3
5
Oleyl Alcohol
4
PEG 16 Lanolin
4
PEG 200 Dilaurate
3
PEG 8 Stearate
3
PG Monostearate
3
PPG 2 Myristyl Propionate
4
Polyglyceryl-3-Diisostearate
4
Potassium Chloride
5

Propylene Glycol Monostearate
4
Red Algae
5
Shark Liver Oil
3
Sodium Chloride (Salt)
5
Sodium Laureth Sulfate
3
Sodium Lauryl Sulfate
5
Solulan 16
4
Sorbitan Oleate
3
Soybean Oil
3
Steareth 10
4
Stearic Acid Tea
3
Stearyl Heptanoate
4
Sulfated Jojoba Oil
3
Stearyl Heptanoate
4

Wheat Germ Glyceride

3

Wheat Germ Oil

5

Xylene

4

TWENTY

JUMPSTART YOUR CLEAR SKIN DIET

To GET YOU started on your new clear skin diet, I've included seven days of delicious, acne-fighting recipes, including seven breakfasts, seven lunches, seven dinners, and a handful of snack ideas. You can find more great acne-friendly recipes on sites like Pinterest by searching key words like antioxidant, vegan, and low-glycemic.

These easy, delicious, superpower meals will start you on your journey to eliminating acne-causing problems with your diet. Feel free to mix and match these recipes and create your own great recipes using ingredients from the lists in chapter nine.

The awesome thing about this diet is that it's not just a clear skin diet. It's an all-over health diet that reduces your risk of cancer, heart attack, and stroke. It increases your energy levels, it's anti-aging, and it'll help you lose weight. What could be better?

Remember, it's not about perfection. If you have to eat meat once a week or you won't even try this diet, then do it. If you go to a birthday party and have a small piece of cake, that doesn't mean you have to start over or chuck the whole thing.

You'll achieve the best results by cutting out dairy, processed foods, and sugar 100%. But you will still see results at a 90% diet—and even 80%. Once I'd been on my own elimination diet for about four months, I could indulge for 10-15% of my weekly meals and keep the improvements in my complexion.

The point is, do your best. Once you start seeing and feeling the results, you'll be hooked.

BREAKFASTS

Banana Orange Delight Smoothie

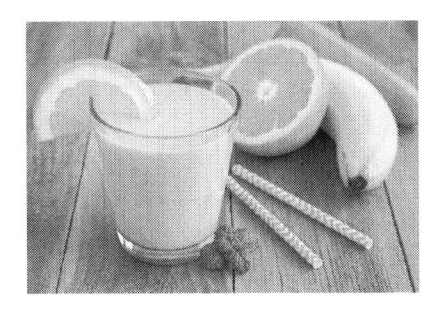

- 3 large carrots, peeled and sliced
- 1 large cucumber, sliced
- 2 oranges, peeled and segmented
- Half a banana, sliced
- Half a can of coconut juice/water (5 ounces)
- ¼ tsp. cinnamon

Blend until the smoothie reaches your desired consistency. Makes two servings.

Chocolate Breakfast Bowl

- 1 cup quinoa
- 1 cup almond milk
- 1 cup coconut milk (from the carton)
- 3 tbsp. unsweetened cocoa powder
- 3 tbsp. maple syrup
- 1/2 tsp. pure vanilla extract
- 4 squares 70% dark chocolate, roughly chopped
- Mixed berries
- Sliced bananas
- Chia seeds

Heat a small saucepan over medium heat. Once hot, add rinsed, drained quinoa and toast for three minutes, stirring frequently.

Add almond milk, coconut milk, and a pinch of salt, and stir. Bring to a boil. Reduce heat to low and simmer for 20-25 minutes, uncovered, stirring occasionally.

Once the liquid is absorbed and the quinoa is tender, remove from heat and add cocoa powder, maple syrup and vanilla. Stir to combine. Taste and adjust flavor as needed.

Serve each bowl of quinoa with a small square of dark chocolate and fresh fruit.

Berry Antioxidant Delight Smoothie

- ½ cup orange juice
- ½ cup seedless grapes
- ½ cup spinach
- ½ cup blueberries
- 1 1/2 tablespoon honey (preferably raw, unfiltered)
- 1 tablespoon flax seeds
- 1 tablespoon oatmeal

Blend ingredients for approximately two minutes. Serve and enjoy!

Pear Toast and Honey

- Rye or barley bread
- 1 pear, sliced thinly
- 1 tbsp. raw, unfiltered honey

Toast the bread. Spread the honey on the toast, and top with the pear slices.

Super Smooth Skin Smoothie

BREAKFASTS

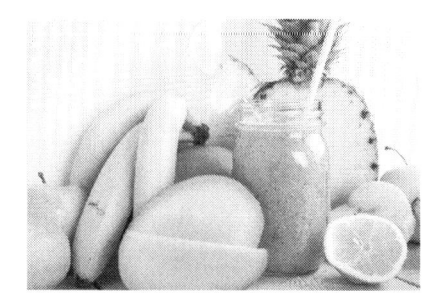

- 1/2 cup coconut water
- 2 frozen bananas, peeled and sliced
- 1 cup chopped pineapple
- 1 cup chopped mango
- 1/2 cup spinach or kale
- 1/2 avocado, sliced
- 3 tbsp. lemon juice

Smoothie on! Yum!

Goji Berry Smoothie

- 1 cup raw spinach or kale
- 1 small apple, sliced
- 1 cup raspberries
- 2 tbsp. goji berries
- 1 tbsp. chia seeds
- 1/2 cup coconut milk

Mix all ingredients in a blender. Serve chilled.

Steel Cut Oats with Nuts and Berries

- 1 cup steel cut oats
- 2 cups almond or coconut milk
- 1/2 cup berries
- 6 walnuts, halved
- ¼ cup almonds
- Pinch of cinnamon to taste

In a saucepan, bring milk to a low boil. Add the oats, reduce heat, and simmer until the oatmeal has soaked in all of the milk and is tender.

Add berries, walnuts, and cinnamon. Serve and enjoy.

LUNCHES

Roasted Tomato and Red Pepper Soup

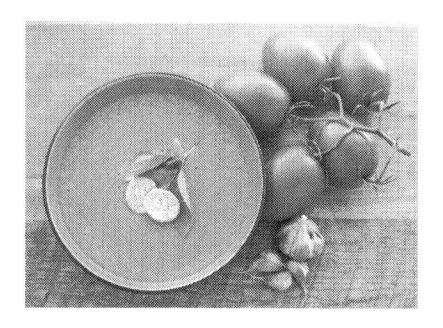

- 8 plum tomatoes, chopped
- 3 red peppers, sliced
- large handful of fresh basil leaves
- handful of fresh rosemary
- bay leaves
- 1 tsp. dried thyme

LUNCHES

- 1/4 cup water
- 3 tsp. apple cider vinegar
- 3 tsp. tomato puree
- Olive oil
- Salt and pepper to taste

Spray a pan with olive oil and place the tomatoes, peppers with the basil leaves, fresh rosemary, dried thyme, bay leaves, salt, and a drizzle more of olive oil on top. Roast at 350 degrees for 30 minutes.

Once veggies are roasted, put them in a blender, or put them in a bowl and use a hand blender. First, add the apple cider vinegar, tomato puree, and salt and pepper. DO NOT add the bay leaves or rosemary sticks.

As the soup blends, slowly add in the water until you reach your desired consistency. Pour and serve.

Quinoa for Clear Skin Salad

- 1 cup quinoa
- 1 1/2 cups water
- 2 cups kale or spinach, chopped
- juice of 1 lemon
- 1/4 cup olive oil
- 1/2 teaspoon salt
- 1 cup pomegranate seeds
- 1/2 cup onion, minced
- 1/4 cup additional olive oil
- 1 avocado, chopped

Cook the quinoa according to box instructions. When cooked, transfer to a large bowl.

In a separate bowl, combine the kale/spinach, lemon juice, olive oil, and salt. Let it wilt for 10 minutes.

When the quinoa has cooled, transfer the kale mixture and mix in the remaining ingredients. Toss well and serve.

Mixed Bean Salad Wrap

- 1 can pinto beans, drained and rinsed
- 1 can kidney beans, drained and rinsed
- ½ cup onion
- ½ cup bell pepper
- 1 tbsp. parsley
- 1 tbsp. lemon juice or mustard
- 1 teaspoon olive oil
- 2 butter lettuce wraps

Combine beans, onions, parsley, bell peppers, lemon juice, and olive oil in a bowl and mix. Scoop evenly into butter lettuce wraps and serve.

Veggie Rainbow Wraps

LUNCHES

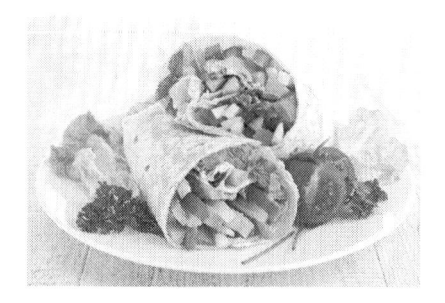

- 2 100% whole wheat wraps
- 1/2 cup diced red pepper
- 1/2 cup diced yellow pepper
- 1/2 cup diced red cabbage
- 2 large carrots, peeled
- 6 - 8 tbsp. hummus
- 2 tbsp. raw sunflower seeds

Heat wraps for 10 to 20 seconds in microwave. Spread each wrap with hummus. Divide veggies and sprinkle on top of the hummus on each wrap.

Make sure to stop the veggies about 2 inches down from the edge of the tortillas to seal them. Starting on the opposite end, roll upwards tightly and press down to seal. Cut like sushi rolls or eat like a wrap.

Roasted Veggies Pita with Sweet Potato Hummus

- 4 whole wheat pitas
- 1 large sweet potatoes
- 1 cup hummus
- 4 cups fresh spinach

- 3 cups chopped butternut squash
- 3 cups mushrooms
- 1 1/2 cups red pepper, chopped
- 1 cup diced red onion
- 1 tbsp. olive oil (or use spray, sparingly)
- 2 tbsp. dried thyme
- 1 tbsp. garlic powder
- Ground black pepper
- 1 cup diced red onion

Preheat oven to 375 degrees. Wash a large sweet potato well, wrap securely with foil. Bake in oven for about 20 - 30 minutes or until fork tender.

In small bowl, mash the sweet potato with fork. Mix together with 1 cup of hummus. Set aside or place in refrigerator.

Arrange the vegetables on a baking sheet and spray or coat with no more than 1 tbsp. of olive oil. Bake at 375 degrees for about 25-35 minutes or till cooked to your preference.

Warm pitas in microwave (20 seconds). Slice pitas in half. Spread each half generously with sweet potato hummus. Stuff each half with 1/2 cup fresh spinach. Add roasted vegetables.

Quinoa Fruit Salad with Honey Vinaigrette

- 1 cup dry quinoa, pre-rinsed
- 2 cups water
- ½ cup strawberries
- ½ cup blueberries
- ½ cup mango chunks

- 2 tbsp. olive oil
- Juice from 1 lime
- 2 tbsp. raw, unfiltered honey

Bring water and quinoa to a boil. Reduce heat to low boil, cover and cook 15 minutes. Turn off heat and let quinoa sit for 5 minutes.

Refrigerate until chilled. Combine the quinoa with the fruit in a bowl. Add olive oil, lime juice, and honey in a bowl and stir well. Toss with the salad and serve.

Avocado Bean Salad

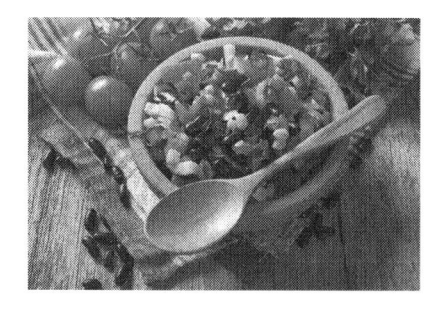

- 1 can (15 oz.) pinto or black beans, rinsed and drained
- 4 tsp. white balsamic vinegar
- 1 avocado, diced
- 2 tsp. fresh lime juice
- 1 cup chopped tomatoes
- 1/2 cup finely chopped red onion
- 1/2 cup finely chopped cilantro

- 1-2 tbsp. olive oil
- Salt and pepper

Blot rinsed beans dry with paper towel, place in plastic bowl, and toss with white balsamic vinegar.

Let beans marinate in the vinegar while you prep other ingredients. Toss avocado in small bowl with lime juice.

Mix onions and cilantro into marinating beans. Use a large spoon to gently fold in avocado and tomato.

Drizzle olive oil over salad and season to taste. Serve immediately at room temperature.

DINNERS

Honey Baked Tofu with Cucumber Salad

- 1 package pressed tofu
- 1 tbsp. cornstarch
- 3 tbsp. honey
- 1 tbsp. soy sauce
- 3 cloves garlic, minced
- Freshly ground pepper, to taste
- Toasted sesame seeds, to garnish
- 1 cup sliced tomatoes
- 1 chopped cucumber
- 1/4 sliced white onion
- 1 sliced green bell pepper
- 1 tsp. olive oil
- Pinch of parsley

Preheat the oven to 400°F. Dry tofu with a paper towel and cut into cubes. Toss with cornstarch and arrange the tofu on a lined baking sheet. Bake for 30-45 minutes. Flip the tofu cubes at midpoint.

A few minutes before baking time is up, start the sauce. In a small frying pan, heat up honey, soy and garlic over medium heat until bubbly and thickened. Season with freshly ground pepper.

Remove the tofu from and toss in the sauce. Garnish with toasted sesame seeds.

For the cucumber salad, combine all ingredients in a bowl. Top with parsley and olive oil. Serve.

Mushroom Burger with Sweet Potato Fries

- 2 large Portobello mushrooms
- 1 red bell pepper, sliced into rings
- ½ red onion, sliced into rings
- 1 cup fresh spinach
- Extra virgin olive oil
- 1 teaspoon dried oregano
- Salt and pepper
- 1 avocado, peeled and pitted
- 3 cloves garlic, peeled
- ¼ cup olive oil
- ¼ cup cilantro leaves
- juice of 1 lemon
- 1 teaspoon red wine vinegar
- Pinch of red chili flakes
- 2 pieces of flatbread pitas or 2 lettuce wraps

- Bag of frozen natural sweet potato fries

Add a drizzle of olive or coconut oil to the grill and bring to medium high heat. Stem the clean Portobello caps and drizzle both sides with olive oil. Season with salt, pepper, and oregano. Grill each side for 10 minutes.

Meanwhile, add a drizzle of olive oil to the red bell pepper and red onion and season with salt and pepper.

Heat a skillet on medium heat and cook the red bell pepper and red onion, stirring occasionally for 10-15 minutes or until softened and lightly browned.

Transfer to a bowl and then add the spinach to the frying pan and cook for 1-2 minutes or until the spinach wilts. Turn off the heat and set aside.

Spoon the avocado into a food processor (or use an immersion blender) with the garlic, olive oil, parsley, cilantro, lemon juice, red wine vinegar, chili flakes, and salt and pepper. Blend for 30 seconds to 1 minute.

Warm the buns or flatbread on the grill or grill pan. Slather the avocado mixture on the bottom bun or piece of flatbread then layer with the mushroom cap, half of the spinach, red bell pepper and onions. Top with the bun and serve with sweet potato fries.

Creamy Cashew and Spinach Noodles

DINNERS

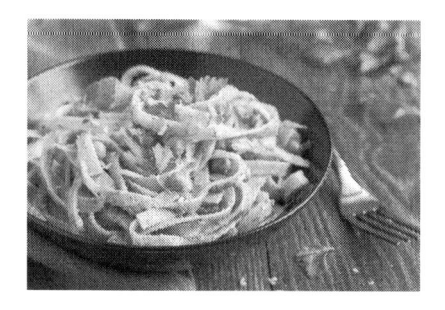

- 1 cup cashews
- ¾ cup water
- ½ teaspoon salt
- 1 clove garlic
- 1 tablespoon oil
- 8 oz. whole wheat fettuccini pasta
- ½ cup cooked peas
- 2 cups baby spinach
- A handful of fresh basil leaves or chives
- Salt and pepper to taste
- Olive oil for drizzling (or coconut oil)

Cover the cashews with water in a bowl and soak for two hours or so. Drain and rinse thoroughly. Place in a food processor or blender (I get better texture with the blender) and add ¾ cup water, salt, and garlic. Puree until very smooth.

Cook pasta until it is al dente. Drain. Heat the oil in a large skillet over medium heat and toss in the spinach - it should wilt pretty quickly.

Add the spinach, peas, half of the herbs, and half of the sauce to the pasta and toss to combine. Add water if the mixture is too sticky. Season with salt and pepper, drizzle with olive oil, and top with the remaining fresh herbs.

Veggie Supreme One-Pot Wonder

- 12 oz. whole wheat linguine, broken in half
- 1 cup packed spinach or kale leaves
- 1 cup chopped roasted red peppers
- 1 can chopped tomatoes, including liquid
- 3-4 large garlic cloves, pressed
- 4 cups vegetable broth
- 2 tablespoons olive oil or coconut oil
- 1 tablespoon kosher salt, plus more to taste
- Pinch red pepper flakes
- Freshly ground black pepper, to taste
- 1 tsp. thyme
- 2 tsp. oregano
- 1 tsp. basil

Combine the first five ingredients in a pot. Next, add the vegetable broth, olive oil, salt, red pepper flakes, black pepper, and other herbs.

Bring your pot to a full rolling boil over high heat. Using tongs, stir and turn the pasta frequently to prevent sticking. Cook until al dente, approximately 9 to 10 minutes.

Remove the pot from heat. The sauce will naturally thicken up after a couple of minutes.

Indian Red Lentil Stew

DINNERS

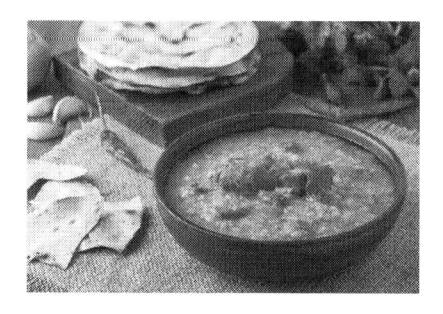

- 1 medium yellow onion, diced
- 2 cups carrots, chopped
- 1 cup celery, chopped
- 2 parsnips, peeled and chopped
- 5 large mushrooms, chopped
- 1 8-oz. can diced tomatoes
- 1/3 cup nutritional yeast
- 1 tbsp. powdered garlic
- 2 tbsp. curry powder
- 2 tbsp. dried dill weed
- 1 tbsp. thyme
- 16 oz. red lentils
- 32 oz. veggie stock

Pour 1 cup of veggie stock into a large stock pot, set on high heat. Add parsnips and water. Sautee on high for 5 minutes. Add carrots and celery and continue to cook on high for another 2 minutes Add onions.

Reduce heat to medium-high. Add red split lentils, onions and allow to cook for 5 minutes over medium-high heat.

Add the rest of your veggie stock and the diced tomatoes and reduce to medium heat. Stir stew well and cook uncovered for 15 minutes, stirring occasionally.

Add mushrooms and spices, stir well and reduce to low heat. Cook an additional 10 minutes, covered.

Delicious Thai Peanut Curry and Rice

- 4 large garlic cloves, minced
- 1/4 cup fresh basil, chopped
- 4 tbsp. chunky peanut butter
- 2 tbsp. curry powder
- 2 cups carrot juice
- 1/2 cup light coconut milk
- 2 tsp. Bragg's Liquid Aminos
- 1 medium red pepper, cut into strips
- 2 cups frozen green beans
- 1 can baby corn
- 3 cups shiitake mushrooms, sliced
- 1/2 eggplant, cubed
- 1 package firm tofu, cubed
- 1/4 cup macadamia nuts, chopped
- 2 tbsp. minced fresh ginger
- Cooked brown or basmati rice

Place the green beans, mushrooms, peppers, corn and eggplant in a sauce pan. Add two cups of carrot juice and the Bragg's Liquid Aminos.

Bring to a boil. Add the garlic, basil, ginger and curry powder. Stir well.

Remove the pan from heat just as the vegetables become cooked through. Remove the vegetables from the juice and reserve the vegetables in a large pot. Put the pan back on medium heat.

Add the peanut butter and coconut milk and stir well to combine. Add the tofu. Cook in the curry sauce for about 10 minutes.

Pour the curry and tofu sauce over the vegetables reserved in the large pot. Stir just to combine (avoid breaking the tofu). Garnish with chopped nuts and basil leaf. Eat as is or serve over brown or basmati rice. Enjoy!

Very Veggie Stir Fry

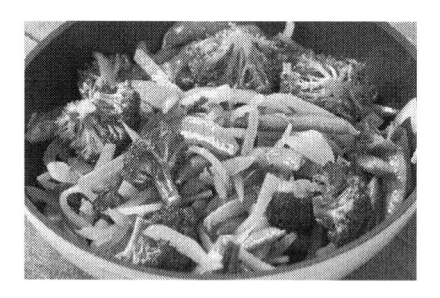

- 2 tablespoons extra light olive oil (or coconut oil)
- 1 red onion, sliced
- 2 cloves garlic, diced
- Sea salt to taste
- 2 cups broccoli florets
- 2 cups yellow and orange peppers, sliced
- 1 cup snow peas
- 5 fresh shiitake mushrooms, sliced

- 1 large bok choy, chopped
- 2 tablespoons plus 1 teaspoon soy sauce
- 2 tablespoons cornstarch
- 1 tablespoon white cooking wine
- 1/2 teaspoon sesame oil
- 1/4 teaspoon rice vinegar
- 1 teaspoon tahini paste
- 1 teaspoon molasses
- 1/8 teaspoon ginger powder
- A pinch of red pepper flakes

Put the onion and garlic, along with the two tablespoons of extra light olive oil and a sprinkle of salt into the frying pan.

Combine the broccoli, cauliflower, carrots and shiitake mushrooms in a large bowl. Keep the bok choy separate.

Turn the frying pan with the onion and garlic to medium high. Stir fry the onions and garlic for about seven minutes, then add the broccoli, cauliflower, carrot and shiitake mushrooms. Stir for five minutes.

In a small bowl, add the soy sauce, corn starch, cooking wine, sesame oil, rice vinegar, tahini, molasses, ginger powder and red pepper flake together. Stir until everything is mixed evenly.

After 5 minutes of cooking the vegetables, add the bok choy and the sauce. Stir fry for 8 minutes, or until the veggies are ready.

SNACKS

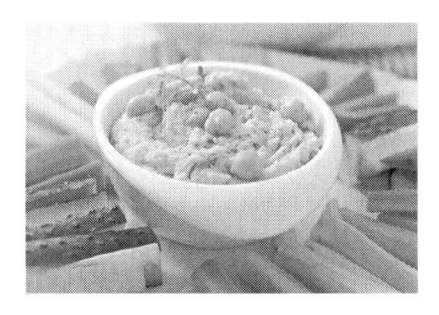

- 1/3 cup dried apricots with almonds
- 1 sliced apple with 2 tablespoons peanut butter
- 1 cup raw veggies with 3 tablespoons hummus
- 1 cup fresh fruit salad with sunflower seeds
- 1 cup sliced veggies with ¼ cup black bean dip
- 1 sliced apple with 1 tbsp. almond butter
- 1 cup celery sticks with 1 tbsp. sugar-free nut butter
- 1 cup steamed edamame
- ½ cup bell pepper slices with ¼ cup hummus

SNACKS

- 2 mandarin oranges
- 1 cup raw veggies with ¼ cup fresh guacamole
- Whole grain tortilla spread with nut butter and sliced banana
- ½ cup baked sweet potato fries
- ½ cup frozen grapes
- ¼ cup dark chocolate-covered almonds
- 8-12 oz. smoothie
- 1 cup berries with cinnamon sprinkles
- ½ cup baked kale chips

ALSO BY KYLA STONE

Beneath the Skin

Before You Break

Rising Storm

Falling Stars

Burning Skies

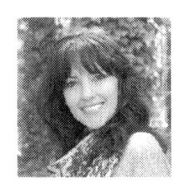

ABOUT THE AUTHOR

KYLA STONE has written for dozens of regional and national publications, including *Pregnancy*, Babble.com, *New York Parenting*, and *Atlanta Parent*.

She lives with her family and two spoiled cats in Atlanta, Georgia. In her free time, she enjoys reading, hiking, photography, and traveling.

Her own twenty-year battle with adult acne inspired her interest in sharing the knowledge that she and others like her have learned in the journey toward clear, healthy skin.

REFERENCES

Amador-Licona N, Diaz-Murillo TA, et al. "Omega-3 Fatty Acids Supplementation and Oxidative Stress in HIV-Seropositive Patients. A Clinical Trial." *Lipids Health Dis.* 2012; 11: 165.

Ballanger F, Baudry P, N'Guyen JM, et al. "Heredity: A Prognostic Factor for Acne." *Dermatology.* 2006; 212: 145-9.

Beeson WL, Mills PK, Phillips RL, Andress M, Fraser GE. "Chronic disease among Seventh-day Adventists, a low-risk group. Rationale, methodology, and description of the population." *Cancer.* 1989; 64: 570–581.

Bernstein CN, Nugent Z, Longobardi T, Blanchard JF. "Isotretinoin is not associated with inflammatory bowel disease:

REFERENCES

a population-based case-control study." *The American journal of gastroenterology.* 2009; 104: 2774-8.

Bershad S. "Developments in topical retinoid therapy for acne." *Semin Cutan Med Surg.* 2001; 20: 154-161.

Bhate K, Williams HC. "Epidemiology of acne vulgaris." *The British journal of dermatology.* 2013; 168: 474-85.

Bhate K, Williams HC. "What's new in acne? An analysis of systematic reviews published in 2011-2012." *Clinical and experimental dermatology.* 2014; 39: 273-7.

Bickers DR, Lim HW, et al. "The burden of skin diseases: 2004 a joint project of the American Academy of Dermatology Association and the Society for Investigative Dermatology." *Journal of the American Academy of Dermatology* 2006; 55: 490-500.

Bowe WP, Joshi SS, Shalita AR. "Diet and acne." *Journal of the American Academy of Dermatology.* 2010; 63: 124-41.

Bowe WP, Logan AC. "Acne vulgaris, probiotics and the gut-brain-skin axis – back to the future?" *Gut Pathog.* 2011 Jan 31; 3(1): 1.

Bowe, Whitney. "Acne vulgaris, probiotics and the gut-brain-skin axis - back to the future?" *Gut Pathog.* 2011; 3: 1. Published online 2011 January 31.

Bowe, Whitney P & Patel, et al. "Acne vulgaris: the role of oxidative stress and the potential therapeutic value of local and systemic antioxidants." *Journal of drugs in dermatology: JDD*, 11. 2012.

Bowe, WP. "Acne vulgaris: the role of oxidative stress and the potential therapeutic value of local and systemic antioxidants." *J Drugs Dermatol.* 2012 Jun; 11(6): 742-6.

Bowe, WP, Joshi SS, et al. "Diet and acne." *J Am Acad Dermatol.* 2010 Jul; 63(1): 124-41.

Chiou WL. "Oral tetracyclines may not be effective in treating acne: dominance of the placebo effect." *Int J Clin Pharmacol Ther.* 2012 Mar; 50(3): 157-61.

Cordain L, Lindeberg S, Hurtado M, et al. "Acne vulgaris: a disease of Western civilization." *Arch Dermatol.* 2002 Dec; 138(12): 1584-90.

Cordain L. "Cereal Grains: Humanity's Double-Edged Sword World." *Rev Nutr Diet.* 1999; 84: 19-73.

Cordain L. "Implications for the role of diet in acne." *Semin Cutan Med Surg.* 2005 Jun; 24(2): 84-91.

Craig W.J. "Nutrition concerns and health effects of vegetarian diets." *Nutr. Clin. Pract.* 2010; 25: 613–620.

REFERENCES

Dall'oglio F, Tedeschi A, Fabbrocini G et al. "Cosmetics for acne: indications & recommendations for an evidence-based approach." *G Ital Dermal Venereol*. 2015; 150(1): 1-11.

Davey GK, Spencer EA, Appleby PN, Allen NE, Knox KH, Key TJ. "EPIC-Oxford: lifestyle characteristics and nutrient intakes in a cohort of 33 883 meat-eaters and 31 546 non meat-eaters in the UK." *Public Health Nutr*. 2003; 6: 259–269.

Dewell A., Weidner G., Sumner M.D., Chi C.S., Ornish D. "A Very-Low-Fat vegan diet increases intake of protective dietary factors and decreases intake of pathogenic dietary factors." *J. Am. Diet. Assoc*. 2008; 108: 347–356.

Draelos ZD. *Atlas of Cosmetic Dermatology*. 1st ed. Philadelphia, Pennsylvania: Churchill Livingstone; 2000.

Ereaux LP. "Facts, fads and fancies in the treatment of acne vulgaris." *Can Med Assoc J*. 1938; 39: 257–61.

Fulton JE Jr, Pay SR, Fulton JEIII. "Comedogenicity of current therapeutic products, cosmetics, ingredients in the rabbit ear." *J Am Acad Dermatol*. 1984; 10: 96-105.

Golandam, Khayef, Young, Julia, et al. "Effects of fish oil supplementation on inflammatory acne." *PLoS One*. 2016 Mar 25; 11: 93.

Golnick H, Cunliffe W, Berson D, et al. "Management of acne: a report from a Global Alliance to Improve Outcomes in Acne." *J Am Acad Dermatol.* 2003; 49: S1–S38.

Goulden V, McGeown CH, Cunliffe WJ. "The familial risk of adult acne: a comparison between first-degree relatives of affected and unaffected individuals." *Br J Dermatol.* 1999; 141: 297-300.

Guarner F, Malagelada JR. "Gut flora in health and disease." *Lancet.* 2003 Feb 8; 361(9356): 512-9.

Guenther LC. "Optimizing treatment with topical tazarotene." *Am J Clin Dermatol.* 2003; 4: 197-202.

Hahm BJ, Min SU, Yoon MY, et al. "Changes of psychiatric parameters and their relationships by oral isotretinoin in acne patients." *The Journal of Dermatology.* 2009; 36: 255-61.

Halder RM, Nootheti PK. "Ethnic skin disorders overview." *J Am Acad Dermatol.* 2003; 48: S143–S148.

Hibbeln JR, Neiminen LR, et al. "Healthy intakes of n–3 and n–6 fatty acids: estimations considering worldwide diversity." *Am J Clin Nutr.* June 2006 vol. 83 no. 6.

Jeremy AH, Holland DB, Roberts SG, et al. "Inflammatory events are involved in acne lesion initiation." *J Invest Dermatol.* 2003; 121: 20–27.

REFERENCES

Jung JY, Yoon MY, Min SU, Hong JS, Choi YS, Suh DH. "The influence of dietary patterns on acne vulgaris in Koreans." *Eur J Dermatol.* 2010; 20: 768–772.

Kaymak Y, Taner E, Taner Y. "Comparison of depression, anxiety and life quality in acne vulgaris patients who were treated with either isotretinoin or topical agents." *International Journal of Dermatology.* 2009; 48: 41-6.

Katsambas A, Papakonstantinou A. "Acne: systemic treatment." *Clinics in Dermatology.* 2004; 22: 412-8.

Kligman AM, Mills OH. "Acne cosmetica." *Arch Dermatol.* 1972; 10:843-50.

Krakowski AC, Eichenfield LF. "Pediatric acne: Clinical presentations, evaluation, and management." *J Drugs Dermatol.* 2007; 6: 589-593.

Layton AM, Morris C, Cunliffe WJ, Ingham E. "Immunohistochemical investigation of evolving inflammation in lesions of acne vulgaris." *Exp Dermatol.* 1998; 7: 191–197.

Logan AC. "Omega-3 Fatty Acids and Acne."*Arch Dermatol.* 2003 Jul; 139(7): 941-2.

Magin P, Pond D, Smith W. "Isotretinoin, depression and suicide: a review of the evidence." *The British journal of general practice: the journal of the Royal College of General Practitioners.* 2005; 55: 134-8.

Marchetti F, Capizzi R, Tulli A. "Efficacy of regulators of the intestinal bacterial flora in the therapy of acne vulgaris." *Clin Ter.* 1987; 122: 339–43.

Marron SE, Tomas-Aragones L, Boira S. "Anxiety, depression, quality of life and patient satisfaction in acne patients treated with oral isotretinoin." *Acta dermato-venereologica.* 2013; 93: 701-6.

Mills. OH, et al. "Comparing 2.5%, 5%, and 10% benzoyl peroxide on inflammatory acne vulgaris." *Int J Dermatol.* 1986 Dec; 25(10): 664-7.

Millikan LE. "The rationale for using a topical retinoid for inflammatory acne." *Am J Clin Dermatol.* 2003; 4: 75-82.

Ozuguz, P, et al. "Evaluation of serum vitamins A and E and zinc levels according to the severity of acne of vulgaris." *Cutan Ocul Toxicol.* 2014 Jun; 33(2): 99-102.

Parodi, A, et al. "Small intestinal bacterial overgrowth in rosacea: clinical effectiveness of its eradication." *Clin Gastroenterol Hepatol.* 2008 Jul; 6(7): 759-64.

Peck GL, Olsen TG, et al. "Isotretinoin versus placebo in the treatment of cystic acne. A randomized double-blind study."

REFERENCES

Journal of the American Academy of Dermatology. 1982; 6: 735-45.

 Plavanich, Molly, Qing Yu Weng, et al. "Low Usefulness of Potassium Monitoring Among Healthy Young Women Taking Spironolactone for Acne." *JAMA Dermatol.* 2015; 151(9): 941-944.

Price, Dr Weston, A. "Nutrition and Physical Degeneration." 6th edition, 14th printing. La Mesa, CA, USA. *Price-Pottenger Nutrition Foundation*, 2000.

Rolewski, S. L. (2003). "Clinical review: topical retinoids". *Dermatology nursing/Dermatology Nurses' Association*, 15(5): 447.

Rubin MG, Kim K, Logan AC. "Acne vulgaris, mental health and omega-3 fatty acids: a report of cases." *Lipids Health Dis.* 2008; 7: 36.

Rubin MG, Kim K, Logan AC. "Acne vulgaris, mental health and omega-3 fatty acids: a report of cases." *Lipids Health Dis* 2008; 7: 36.

Schaefer O. "When the Eskimo comes to town." *Nutr Today.* 1971; 68-16.

Simonart T. "Newer approaches to the treatment of acne vulgaris." *American Journal of Clinical Dermatology.* 2012; 13: 357-64.

REFERENCES

Siver RH. "Lactobacillus for the control of acne." *J Med Soc New Jersey*. 1961; 59: 52–53.

Smith RN, Mann NJ, Braue A, et al. "A low-glycemic-load diet improves symptoms in acne vulgaris patients: a randomized controlled trial." *Am J Clin Nutr*. 2007 Jul; 86(1): 107-15.

Smith RN, Mann NJ, Braue A, Makelainen H, Varigos GA. "The effect of a high-protein, low glycemic-load diet versus a conventional, high glycemic-load diet on biochemical parameters associated with acne vulgaris: a randomized, investigator-masked, controlled trial." *J Am Acad Dermatol*. 2007; 57: 247–256.

Smith EV, Grindlay DJ, Williams HC. "What's new in acne? An analysis of systematic reviews published in 2009-2010." *Clin Exp Dermatol*. 2011; 36(2): 119-22; quiz 123.

Smith RN, Braue A, Varigos GA, Mann NJ. "The effect of a low glycemic load diet on acne vulgaris and the fatty acid composition of skin surface triglycerides." *J Dermatol Sci*. 2008; 50: 41–52.

Spencer EH, Ferdowsian HR, Barnard ND. "Diet and acne: a review of the evidence." *Int J Dermatol*. 2009 Apr; 48(4): 339-47.

Strauss JS, Krowchuk DP, Leyden JJ, et al. "Guidelines of care

REFERENCES

for acne vulgaris management." *Journal of the American Academy of Dermatology*. 2007; 56: 651-63.

T.J. Rogers, E. Balish. "Immunity to Candida Albicans Microbiol." *Rev*. 1980, 44(4): 660.

Thiboutot DM, Strauss JS. "Diet and Acne Revisited." *Arch Dermatol*. 2002 Dec; 138(12): 1591-2.

Tobechi L., Ebede, MD, et al. "Hormonal Treatment of Acne in Women." *J Clin Aesthet Dermatol*. 2009 Dec; 2(12): 16–22.

Veith WB, Silverberg NB. "The association of acne vulgaris with diet." *Cutis*. 2011 Aug; 88(2): 84-91.

Verallo-Rowell VM. "The validated hypoallergenic cosmetics rating system: its 30–year evolution and effect on the prevalence of cosmetic reactions." *Dermatitis*. 2011; 22(2): 80-97.

Walton S, Wyatt EH, Cunliffe WJ. "Genetic control of sebum excretion and acne—a twin study." *Br J Dermatol*. 1988 Mar; 118(3): 393-6.

Williams HC, Dellavalle RP, Garner "S. Acne vulgaris." *Lancet*. 2012; 379(9813): 361-72.

Wolverton SE, Harper JC. "Important controversies associated with isotretinoin therapy for acne." *American Journal of Clinical Dermatology*. 2013; 14: 71-6.

Yesilova Y, Bez Y, Ari M, Kaya MC, Alpak G. "Effects of isotretinoin on obsessive compulsive symptoms, depression, and anxiety in patients with acne vulgaris." *The Journal of Dermatological Treatment.* 2012; 23: 268-71.

Zhang H, Liao W, Chao W, et al. "Risk factors for sebaceous gland diseases and their relationship to gastrointestinal dysfunction in Han adolescents." *J Dermatol.* 2008 Sep; 35(9): 555-61.

Zhang H, Liao W, et al. "Risk factors for sebaceous gland diseases and their relationship to gastrointestinal dysfunction in Han adolescents." *J Dermatol.* 2008; 35: 555–61.

Printed in Poland
by Amazon Fulfillment
Poland Sp. z o.o., Wrocław